Between Therapist and Client

A Series of Books in Psychology

Editors:
Richard C. Atkinson
Gardner Lindzey
Richard F. Thompson

Between Therapist and Client
The New Relationship

Michael Kahn

W. H. Freeman and Company
New York

Library of Congress Cataloging-in-Publication Data

Kahn, Michael D., 1936-
    Between therapist and client : the new relationship /
Michael Kahn.
        p.   cm. — (A series of books in psychology)
    Includes bibliographical references and index.
    ISBN 0-7167-2178-3   ISBN 0-7167-2194-5 (pbk.)
    1. Psychotherapist and patient.   2. Psychotherapy.   I.
Title.   II. Series.
    RC480.8.K34   1991
    616.89′14 — dc20   90-48791
                                                            CIP

Printed in the United States of America

1 2 3 4 5 6 7 8 9 0   VB   9 9 8 7 6 5 4 3 2 1 0

To my father, John Tuteur, Sr.

Contents

Preface

In a J. D. Salinger story, the young author, Buddy Glass, receives this advice from his older brother:

> Remember before ever you sit down to write that you've been a *reader* long before you were ever a writer. You simply fix that fact in your mind, then sit very still and ask yourself, as a reader, what piece of writing in all the world Buddy Glass would most want to read if he had his heart's choice. The next step is . . . you just sit down shamelessly and write the thing yourself.[1]

I've been a client long before I ever was a therapist. This book is about the way I would like a therapist to be with me if I had my heart's choice.

The subtitle, "The New Relationship," has, as I hope will become clear, two meanings. First, it means that in the field of psychotherapy, the beginnings of reconciliation between previously competing traditions open new possibilities for the way therapists relate to clients. Second, it means that in successful therapy the therapist provides for the client a relationship unlike any the client has had before.

For some time it has seemed to me that the training of psychotherapists would be helped by a book that brought together two major therapeutic traditions that have been separated through a series of sociological accidents. The two traditions are the humanistic psychologist's concern for a warm and empathic clinical relationship and the psychoanalyst's interest in bringing to the surface the unconscious aspects of that relationship, that is, the phenomena of transference and countertransference.

For several years I taught a course that attempted to explore the possibilities of that integration; this book is the outgrowth of that course. I hope that it will prove useful to student therapists trying to keep their bearings on what can be turbulent and very confusing seas. I hope that it might also be useful to practicing therapists who may not have had time to keep up with some of the most interesting recent developments in contemporary thinking about the clinical relationship. And though it is addressed to therapists, it would give me pleasure if people who are not practicing clinicians found the book interesting. I have tried to make it accessible to them, as well as to therapists.

The book contains many brief clinical illustrations. In most places, I have indicated which of these are taken from my own practice and which are borrowed from other authors. Where neither of those attributions appear, the illustration has been invented, although probably none of them is *truly* invented. It's just that I no longer remember which client taught them to me.

Many people have helped me in the course of writing this book. My (very) significant other, Virginia Stutcki, and my colleagues Jeff Shapiro and Brant Cortright read the entire manuscript chapter by chapter, and, in addition to making invaluable suggestions, gave me support and encouragement. My editor, Jonathan Cobb, has been a good deal more than that. He has been a skillful and gentle writing teacher and a supportive friend. Diane Maass, my project editor, lovingly saw the book through from manuscript to completion, proofread it, and saw to its visual aesthetics. My colleagues Karen Peoples, Bill Littlewood, Dean Elias, and Jacqueline West gave me significant assistance on one or more chapters. Donald P. Spence and Dale G. Larson read an early version of the manuscript and made valuable suggestions. Harvey Peskin graciously helped me purge the book of the most glaring of my prejudices. My brother, John Tuteur, an English scholar, persuaded me to excise about half of the adjectives and adverbs. The reader will have cause to thank him. My friend and colleague Jack Clareman has supported me through the writing of this book in more ways than I can name. And like most teachers and therapists, I am aware that much of what I know, I have learned from my students and my clients. My thanks to all.

Michael Kahn
August, 1990

I

Why Study the Relationship?

When I was a graduate student, I once asked a teacher of mine, a therapist of many years' experience, if he got bored doing clinical work. He thought it over and then replied that he'd been bored infrequently. "The more I've learned about the relationship, the more interesting the work has become," he said.

"The *relationship*?" I asked.

"I think so," he said. "It seems there are long periods when nothing very new is revealed about the client's symptoms or his history. But that certainly isn't true about the relationship. I think I learn more about that every year, and the more I learn, the more it keeps me on my toes. There is so much going on every minute, I can't possibly stay with it all, and sometimes it goes so fast that I'm busy figuring out what I want to do about it. All of that seems so interesting, it would be hard to get bored."

"But why so much attention to the relationship?" I asked.

He looked puzzled for a moment. "Because the relationship *is* the therapy," he said.

Now *I* was puzzled. I was at the time deeply immersed in learning about analytic insights and how they are discovered and revealed to the client. I told him that and said I thought *that* was the therapy.

"Insight is important," he said. "But it's certainly not enough. I think the future lies in understanding the nature of the relationship between the therapist and the client."

That was more than thirty years ago, and I have come to believe that he was ahead of his time. I think he was right that the therapist – client relationship itself holds enormous therapeutic potential, and I have discovered that he was also right that attending to that relationship can be immensely interesting.

In this book I will suggest some ways to look at the clinical relationship and some actions that the therapist can take to help the client as the relationship develops. I'm going to do that by looking at how some of the important thinkers in our field have variously conceptualized the relationship and how they have advised us to deal with it. Then I will offer a synthesis of those points of view to provide the therapist with some useful guidelines for working with clients.

There are two main reasons for making a careful study of the clinical relationship. First, it is risky not to. Much that transpires between therapist and client is subtle indeed. And subtle or not, each small vagary is likely to be charged with extreme importance for the client. The therapy and even the client can be damaged when the therapist is insufficiently aware of how easy it is to get into trouble.

Most beginning clinicians understand that it is important to live by the basic ground rules of therapy. Confidentiality must be honored, and the boundaries of the therapeutic relationship must be respected, which means remembering every moment that our clients are neither friends nor lovers. Most therapists know these rules, but until one has grasped just how subtle and complex the relationship can be, and how important the therapist becomes to the client, one is likely to seriously underestimate how easy it is to damage the therapy. The slightest breach of confidentiality can be magnified by the client into a major betrayal; a chance encounter with a client outside the consulting room can evolve into a problematic social situation and have serious repercussions. An offhand remark or thoughtless joke can cause pain or confusion the client may not be able to acknowledge. None of these slips is likely to cause irreparable harm, but a sophisticated alertness to the vagaries of the relationship will minimize the chances of such slips occurring and will put the therapist in a stronger position to rectify the oversights should they occur.

The second reason for attending to the relationship is that it gives one a major therapeutic advantage. This book will take the position that awareness of the subtleties and changes in the relationship provides the therapist with a powerful tool, perhaps the most powerful therapeutic tool of all. It will try to show why that is true and how that tool might be used in our work with clients.

In psychodynamic therapy, which includes the various psychoanalytic-based therapies (including, or course, self-psychology), object-relations therapies, Gestalt therapies, and various body-oriented therapies, awareness of the relationship is an indispensable tool. And even those who choose not to deal explicitly with the relationship, such as behavior therapists, cognitive therapists, and advice-giving counselors, will avoid a good many pitfalls if they are sophisticated about what might happen in the relationship between therapist and client.

Five Propositions

This, then, is a book about understanding and dealing with the clinical relationship. It is built around the following propositions.

1. Insight is not enough. Even many years after the early clinicians discovered this, I suppose most therapists still experience (at least occasionally) the frustration and disappointment of uncovering and conveying a really *good* insight, only to discover it didn't prompt much change in the client. Insight is necessary — but not sufficient.

2. The ingredient that needs to be added to insight is an *understanding* of the nature of the relationship and the way the therapist deals with it. Practically all schools of therapy agree that this understanding is needed. When they do disagree, it is over the *nature* of that relationship and how it should be dealt with by the therapist.

3. One of the reasons the therapist–client relationship has such therapeutic potential, is that it is the one relationship in the client's life that is actually happening during the therapy hour. During that time all other relationships are more abstract, more distant.

4. There was a time when selecting a training program meant choosing between a program that taught you how to understand the relationship and one that encouraged you to develop an accepting warmth toward the client. It was hard to find one that did both. The programs that emphasized the relationship also encouraged the therapist to adopt a stance of cool, distant "neutrality," so as not to influence the developing relationship. This meant that only those therapists studying in programs with a

heavily psychoanalytic emphasis were taught very much about either the subtle complexities of the therapeutic relationship or the ways it might be handled for the benefit of the client.

5. In recent years, however, there has been a marked rapprochement between those who understand and work with the complexities of the relationship and those who understand the necessity of that relationship's being warm and humane. A student no longer has to choose between the two.

A Short History of the Relationship

It will add perspective to our explorations to take a brief look at the history of how our profession has regarded the clinical relationship. Then in the following chapters we'll look in more detail at the ideas of Sigmund Freud, Carl Rogers, Merton Gill, and Heinz Kohut, as we begin to construct a way of using the relationship in the practice of psychotherapy.

The Freudian beginnings

It is important to remember that psychotherapy began as a medical specialty. Physicians, particularly nineteenth-century physicians, were trained to believe that what mattered was what you *did* to and for the patient; the relationship itself, sometimes contemptuously dismissed as "bedside manner," was considered irrelevant. Sigmund Freud and his coworker Joseph Breuer[1] were physicians, with the attitude and assumptions that implied. In their early work together, in the 1880s and 1890s, they were trying to cure the condition called *hysteria* by figuring out what to *do* — that is, how to *treat* the condition as you would treat any disease. In the next chapter, we will follow Freud's path from a no-nonsense medical stance to an ever-growing conviction that the relationship between analyst and patient* was crucial, that it was invariably intense, mysterious, and very complex, however it might appear on the surface. As we will see, this view of the clinical relationship included the remarkable observation that patients *transfer* onto the therapist their attitudes, feelings, fears, and wishes from long ago. Freud came to believe it essential that the therapist recognize this *transference* and know how to respond to it. He believed it had the power to hinder or further the treatment, depending on how it was dealt with. Eventually he saw the transference as the therapist's central opportunity and main point of therapeutic leverage.

In the 70 years following Freud's early work with transference, this line of thought underwent some dramatic developments. Freud's way of being with his patients was active and engaged. As he reports it in his published case studies,[2,3] his approach was very different from the picture we have today of the silent, detached analyst. Sometimes he talked as much as the patient, carrying on a real dialogue. If a patient was hungry, he might feed him. To support one of his patients he took up an annual collection of money from his psychoanalytic colleagues. And so on.

The early analysts, following much of what Freud preached, if not what he practiced, believed that the best service they could render their patients was to get out of the

---

*I prefer the word *client* to *patient* since I see the people with whom I work, not as sick, but rather as people with problems like my own, trying to grow as I am trying to grow. I will use "patient" when discussing Freud's beliefs, since his model was so markedly doctor–patient. Elsewhere I will use "client".

way as much as possible. They sat out of sight, and much of the time they kept quiet. They had three reasons for this approach.

First, they believed, following Freud, that the patient's difficulty came primarily from internal psychic conflict: conflict between wish and fear, conflict between incompatible wishes. If, then, they managed to keep quiet, and let the patients find their way into the expression of their deepest wishes and fears, those conflicts would emerge from the unconscious into the light of day. Once made conscious, those deep impulses and anxieties would have less power to dominate the patient.

Second, they believed that the transference would develop most fully if the analyst were a "blank screen" onto which the transference phenomena could be projected. Being a blank screen meant staying quiet and staying out of the way as much as possible, thus furnishing minimal cues about the actuality of the analyst's person.

Third, they believed that, for therapy to progress, the analytic process required "optimal frustration." Thus the analyst seldom responded directly to the patient. In fact, the ideal was *never* to respond directly to the patient. Questions were not answered, pleasantries were not returned, compliments were not acknowledged, and accusations were not countered. The rule was, "The analyst gives the patient *nothing* but interpretations." Analysts readily acknowledged that this was a frustrating situation for the patient. Say "Good morning," and get nothing back but silence. Ask a question about what that last interpretation meant, and hear only silence. Tell your analyst you're really angry, and get no response. The early analysts believed the frustration thus evoked in their patients was the energizer that stirred inner conflicts and caused them to emerge from the depths.

As analysts gained experience with this way of working, it became clear to the most sensitive of them that if they were going to practice this highly disciplined approach to therapy, they would have to do it in the context of a great deal of loving compassion. Otherwise the relationship would be perceived by the patient as sadistic dominance. It's not easy to communicate loving compassion when your rules allow you to give nothing but interpretation. It probably can be done, but it takes a person of unusually large heart and unusually well-developed communication skills. Freud himself seldom attempted it. He permitted himself a good deal of active engagement with his patients, whether or not that clashed with his beliefs.

So, theoretically, there were two possible ways of being truly therapeutic: One could be considerably more engaged with one's patients than the rules permitted, or one could be an unusually warm and compassionate person with an unusual capacity to communicate that compassion. Actually, I believe, the analysts were caught in an impossible contradiction. On the one hand, they required of themselves that they maintain a relatively severe neutrality, and on the other hand, they needed to create a therapeutic ambience of trust, security, and confidence.

What happened all too often was that the analyst became the deadpan, silence-at-all-costs modern psychoanalyst, ripe for parody. In her book *The Impossible Profession* Janet Malcolm relates the famous story of the patient who came to a session on crutches and swathed in bandages. The analyst, a consummate professional, said nothing, merely sat stonily and waited for the associations to begin.

It is crucial to note here that when the psychoanalysts speak of being *neutral*, they do not mean being cold and inhuman. Neutrality implies keeping a respectful distance so that patients can find their own way and so the analyst's ideas are not imposed upon them. It means respecting the patient's autonomy and integrity. It means allowing patients to set and to change the emotional tone of the relationship. It also means giving them confidence that you will offer consistency no matter what they do. That this honorable concept has led some analysts to act coldly to their patients should in no way detract from its power and its usefulness. It remains a valuable concept.

Extreme nonresponsiveness has for some years been under increasing criticism from all sides. Many contemporary psychoanalysts find it countertherapeutic. And to most therapists trained outside the analytic institutes (and many inside) it seems ethically and humanly unacceptable.

At its worst, nonresponsiveness is seen by the client as hostility. Even at its best, unless the analyst is a truly remarkable human being, it's hard to imagine that the cause of human growth is served by such a cold and manifestly inhumane relationship. The early analysts have much to teach us about the clinical relationship (after all, they invented the subject), and we will do well to ponder their insights carefully. But fewer and fewer analysts themselves any longer believe in the cool, nonresponsive stance.

Carl Rogers and the humanistic revolution

The field of therapy was dominated by the psychoanalysts until the 1940s when an American psychologist named Carl Rogers sounded a decidedly American response to this European therapy.[4] As we will see in Chapter 3, his view of the clinical relationship was very different from that of the analysts, and it became hugely popular in the ensuing 30 years, particularly in the United States. Though there are probably fewer pure Rogerians practicing today than 20 years ago, Rogers' influence is still widespread and

9

constitutes a major force in contemporary American thinking about psychotherapy.

The clinical relationship that Rogers proposed was radically different from the nonresponsiveness that had come to predominate in American psychoanalysis. He taught that the therapeutic attitude required *empathy* and *unconditional positive regard* for the client and *genuineness* on the part of the therapist. Although the psychoanalytic influence remained strong in American clinics, the clients of an increasing number of psychologists and other counselors began to be treated in a much more human, and perhaps humane, fashion than were the patients of many of the analysts.

The revolution of the 1960s

As it did on all aspects of American life, the 1960s had a profound effect on psychotherapy. For one thing, Rogers' influence became significantly alloyed by two forces of the sixties. The first was the political climate. To the radical consciousness of the sixties, the undemocratic psychoanalytic relationship was an anathema relying, as it did, on a severe power imbalance between therapist and client. Two of Rogers' main tenets, uncompromising respect for his clients and a firm refusal to impose interpretations upon them, made his approach less objectionable to this political consciousness. Nonetheless, even in Rogers' method the power imbalance remained: Self-revelation was expected of the client, whereas the therapist, however warm and respectful, remained hidden. Therapists influenced by radical politics searched for ways to make the clinical relationship even more egalitarian than Rogers had done.

The second significant force of the sixties was the *encounter* movement of the newly popular humanistic psychology.[5] This tradition emphasized *authenticity* and *sym-*
10

metry. Authenticity implied that the therapist should be as honest and as emotionally exposed as the client, and symmetry, echoing the politics of the day, demanded that the therapist be willing to do anything the client was asked to do. It's not clear whether Rogers understood *genuineness* to mean the same thing that the encounter psychologists meant by *authenticity*, but there is no doubt that in practice they were very different. Rogers and his students practiced genuineness in the context of gentleness and positive regard. The encounter people tended to view authenticity in a context of unrestrained confrontation; for them, what was therapeutic was the participation in an authentic relationship, "authentic" meaning that therapists would openly share whatever feelings were stirred in them by their clients. Hostility, boredom, excitement, sexual attraction, any feeling might be expressed; what mattered was the honest sharing.

Rogers was actively involved in the encounter movement and considered himself importantly influenced by it. Nonetheless, just as his concept of genuineness was practiced by others in a context very different from his own, his notion of positive regard was taken to extremes that he had almost certainly not intended: Psychologists influenced by sixties viewpoints saw their mission as giving the client considerable, often physical, loving support, sometimes laced with confrontation. This kind of clinical relationship has flourished over the past 20 years.

The psychoanalysts respond

It could be expected that many psychoanalysts would be critical of these trends, and indeed they were. First, they were concerned that the new therapeutic style was extremely confusing to the client, who might well wonder

11

whether the person sitting opposite was therapist, friend, or antagonist. And just whose needs was the therapist there to serve, anyway?

Second, they worried that, freed to follow any impulse, there would be little to prevent the therapist from acting out the deepest countertransference feelings and thus severely exploiting the client. *Countertransference*, which we will examine in detail in Chapter 6, was Freud's term for the unconscious feelings stirred in the analyst by the patient. The patient, Freud taught, can stimulate in the analyst strong needs to act out old dramas and to gratify old unsatisfied needs. The analyst was to protect the patient by unremitting vigilance against these impulses. "Authenticity" looked to the analysts like a license to carry and use dangerous weapons.

Third, they saw no way that the patient's transference could be understood and utilized if it were so hopelessly confounded by the freely expressed reality of the therapist's personality.

Finally, the sixties trends in clinical practice caused a crucial issue to be joined: Should the client be gratified or frustrated? The analysts held a firm position that frustration is necessary to the therapeutic process. Their argument went like this: all humans are irresistibly drawn to gratification and can't be expected to choose hard work when gratification seems to be offered free (few people would dig ditches if the same salary were offered for doing nothing); in fact, however, the gratification offered in the therapist's office is illusory. It is built on the denial of great human truths: We are alone, we are mortal, we are imperfect, and the world around us is, if anything, even more imperfect. There are no free lunches and few affordable ones.

The analysts believe that to learn these lessons the childhood illusions of merger and bliss must be analyzed and laid to rest. Then the hard truths of self-reliance can be accepted and the person can seek real, if limited, gratifications, rather than illusions, which will vanish as he walks out of the therapist's office. Gratifications offered by the therapist merely prolong the illusion that the ultimate gratifier is out there somewhere if only one keeps searching.

I hardly need point out how radically different this view of reality is from the sunny optimism of Carl Rogers and the American humanists.

A period of controversy

Thus our field emerged from the sixties in a state of sharp controversy. Should we be warm or neutral? Should we lay back, or should we mix it up? Should we frustrate or gratify? Should we keep the boundaries of the relationship very strict, or should we chat with our clients, socialize with them, and make friends of them? And perhaps the most important controversy of all, are we to discuss with clients their relationship with us? Is it important that they tell us their feelings about us? Is it important that we search for feelings about us that they're not telling? For some years it seemed that there were persuasive advocates at both extremes and not very many trying to thread their way down the center.

From an unexpected source: rapprochement

And then from within the psychoanalytic movement itself, from the very heart of the psychoanalytic establishment, a new set of voices began to be heard. Two of the most articulate and comprehensive of these voices are those of Heinz Kohut[6] and Merton Gill.[7] Kohut argued persuasively that the cold, unyielding stance of some contempo-

13

rary analysts was seen by the client as the most painful and destructive sort of rejection. This was just the sort of rejection from the client's family that had gotten the client into trouble in the first place. Trying to cure it with more of the same was like pouring gasoline onto the fire. Just as Rogers had talked of the central importance of empathy, Kohut, from inside the psychoanalytic movement, in fact as a past president of the prestigious American Psychoanalytic Association, was now speaking of visible, demonstrated empathy as one of the most important qualities the therapist had to offer the client.

Meanwhile, Merton Gill, another therapist with impeccable psychoanalytic credentials, was pointing out the striking difference between the cool stance of some modern analysts and Freud's warm interactions with his patients. Gill reminded his colleagues that human civility was an important part of the analytic ambience.

In spite of the similarities to Roger's advocacy of warmth, neither Gill nor Kohut had become Rogerians. Rogers had placed no particular importance on encouraging the client to attend to and discuss the relationship with the therapist, nor had he given any weight to consideration of the unconscious. Gill and Kohut, on the other hand, were both psychoanalysts. Their therapies were built around the conception of the unconscious, and they held fast to the psychoanalytic notion that *working with the relationship* between therapist and client was of central importance. We will see in the chapters ahead how each of them interpreted that concept and how similar many of their ideas are. For now, it is enough to note that they have introduced a hugely important middle way between the schools of warm support and those of neutral transference analysis, a middle way that combines the advantages of warm engagement

with the advantages of working actively with the relationship itself.

The sine qua non: nondefensiveness

These two pioneers, as we will see, also added another
major component to the kind of therapy they developed.
Though they use different vocabularies, it is clear that each
of them considers crucial the attribute of *nondefensiveness.*
To Kohut, this attribute provides the essential context for
the kind of interpretation and analysis necessary for successful therapy. But to Gill, this attribute of nondefensiveness is
what actually effects the therapy. Gill teaches that, beginning with our parents, we encounter people throughout our
lives who have so much to defend that we learn, at worst, to
keep our feelings to ourselves or, at best, to expect the
expression of those feelings to be met with little more than
a defensive riposte. This is not a criticism of the socializing
community; it's just the way it is. The therapeutic relationship is crucially different in that expressed feelings about
the therapist are not met with a defensive countermove, but
rather with warm encouragement to explore them further.
This is a remarkable combining of the Freudian concern
with the relationship and the Rogerian emphasis on
warmth and support. And as such, it, together with Kohut's
insights, opens a whole new path for the clinician.

It has probably occurred to you that nondefensiveness is a
good deal easier to prescribe than to practice. When threatened in any way, the temptation to fight back, to explain, to
justify, to one-up, to go coldly silent is almost overwhelming in all but saints, and there are few saints in our profession. Yet I hope you will find that once nondefensiveness is
made an explicit goal and a manageable technique, once

you have seen the enormous value it offers clients, you will find it increasingly possible to follow Kohut and Gill into this threatening, enormously fascinating, and fruitful realm.

Existential psychology

There is one other therapeutic tradition that deserves mention — existential psychology. Growing out of European existentialism, it flowered in America in the late 1950s and had a clear influence on the humanistic psychology of the 1960s. We will not examine it separately because its view of the clinical relationship is close to those encountered in the authors we will study. But as a part of the humanistic psychology movement it has had a great impact and thus deserves mention in this historical survey.

Rollo May, perhaps the most articulate and influential of the American existential psychotherapists, once said that he hoped there would never be a school of existential psychotherapy, but rather that the insights of the existentialists would permeate all schools. He gives what is perhaps one of his central insights in his paper "The Emergence of Existential Psychology":

> There is no such thing as truth or reality for a living human being except as he participates in it, is conscious of it, has some relationship to it. We can demonstrate at every moment of the day in our psychotherapeutic work that only the truth that comes alive, becomes more than an abstract ideal but is "felt on the pulse," only the truth that is genuinely experienced on all levels of being, . . . only this truth has the power to change a human being.[8]

An abstract discussion of the client's problems or history is not likely to produce much change. Existential therapy is sometimes called *Dasein* analysis. *Dasein* roughly translates "being there." The idea, of course, is that therapy works when the client is really *there*, rather than merely talking about herself — a view that is shared by Rogers, Gill, and Kohut.

From Dilemma to Dialectic

The old dilemmas that asked the clinician to choose between empathic warmth and active exploration of the relationship are being transformed by modern workers into dialectic, raising the possibility of a new synthesis. In the chapters that follow we will look at this transformation in detail and then describe the emerging synthesis, as well as the clinical style and technique it implies.

Though it may sound as if I think that all the dilemmas have now been resolved, I am not so naive. The great questions of psychotherapy will never be definitively answered. Nonetheless, some interesting congruences are beginning to appear in the field. In spite of continuing sharp controversies and differences even among sympathetic colleagues, there is a growing unity of thought about ways of dealing with these issues in therapy. And these congruences can provide a useful set of guidelines for a beginning therapist. Every therapist eventually puts together his or her own method, but one needs to start somewhere. This book will suggest a place to start.

2

The Discovery of Transference

SIGMUND FREUD

Not long ago, teaching the ideas of Sigmund Freud to graduate students was an exercise in diplomacy and public relations. Freud was definitely "out," and it took some doing to get students even to consider that he might be worth reading. Feminists were understandably concerned about the nineteenth-century Germanic sexism in his writing. Humanistic psychologists found him gloomy and discouraging, in sharp contrast to the optimism they were trying to promulgate. They also objected to his view of human beings as merely the highest form of animal, fearing that he omitted the spiritual, transcendent nature of the human being. Radicals found him authoritarian and disapproved of the power imbalance between analyst and patient.

One consequence of these reactions was that the Freudian insights disappeared from much of the clinical training outside the psychoanalytic institutes. It was as though English departments had stopped teaching Shakespeare because of his anti-Semitism or mathematics departments had suppressed Einstein because of his part in the chain of discoveries leading to the atom bomb.

Now all that is rapidly changing. There remains some residual prejudice against Freud, but it has greatly lessened, and the field of clinical practice is in a position to study his work more objectively, taking from it what is useful. There are influential feminist sociologists and psychologists, such as Nancy Chodorow,[1,2] who consider themselves Freudians and are attempting to integrate Freudian thought into the new political awareness. Many in the feminist movement are coming to believe that it is difficult to understand the causes and effects of sexism — or for that matter, to understand the human mind — without the illumination of Freud's theory of the unconscious.

As we will see in subsequent chapters, the humanistic tradition is at last finding avenues of rapprochement with psychoanalysis. And as 1960s radicalism has softened during the past ten years, politically conscious psychologists have come to look for ways to make psychotherapy more egalitarian without discarding the most valuable contributions of psychoanalysis.

All of these changes have reduced the antipathy to Freud and made it possible once again to incorporate his insights into the development of modern psychotherapy.

In the 50 years since Freud's death, psychology has moved on, building on his and his colleagues' work, developing theories of clinical practice more sophisticated and more effective than the psychoanalysis he left us. Nonetheless, he is the most powerful, original, and influential writer psychology has produced; studying the mind without studying Freud is like studying evolution without Darwin.

It is not just the psychologist who is limited by ignoring Freudian theory; it is all of us. Freud cast a light deep into the hidden recesses of the mind, making visible a vast new world. Our view of ourselves and others is made infinitely richer (if sometimes more unsettling) by that illumination. For therapists, part of that richness is what we can now recognize in our relationships with clients. Freud taught us how to see the remarkable drama taking place in the consulting room.

Let's look at how that came about.

Breuer and Bertha: The Discovery of Transference

At the very beginning of his career Freud witnessed a remarkable event. His friend and mentor, Josef Breuer, was treating an attractive young woman for hysteria. He saw this woman, whose name was Bertha, twice a day, often in her bedroom. He talked about her constantly. It was clear to Freud that Breuer was fascinated with Bertha. And it shortly became clear to him that the fascination was by no means one-way. Breuer was summoned to the house one evening to find Bertha in great distress. She announced to him that she was pregnant with his child. Of course, Breuer knew that their relationship had been impeccably ethical; moreover, he was convinced that she was a virgin. And, indeed, the "pregnancy" turned out to be entirely hysterical.

In Chapter 1 we noted that Freud, a nineteenth-century physician, had begun with a very mechanical view of the therapeutic relationship. Observing what had happened between Breuer and his patient, he began to understand that the therapeutic relationship was much deeper and more complex than that described in the conventional view of the doctor – patient relationship. For the rest of his life he struggled to understand the nature of the therapist – patient relationship and how it could best be dealt with. To increase his understanding he looked to his most important source of information: his own and his colleagues' patients. As he scrutinized those relationships there emerged two discoveries that will particularly concern us.

The Theory of Templates

In our earliest relationships we establish templates, patterns into which we tend to fit all of our subsequent relationships or at least all of our *important* subsequent relationships.[3] If I had a warm and supportive relationship with my father, it is likely that I will tend to see male authority figures in a positive light. I will seek out that kind of relationship, will expect good things from it, and will behave in ways to maximize the chance that it will indeed turn out well. If, on the other hand, my father was particularly critical of me, it is likely that I will tend to see men in authority as critical and to relate to them in that way. If I had to struggle with my siblings for parental attention, it is probable that I will see peers as competitors for scarce resources. And so on.

The spoken associations of Breuer's patient Bertha led Freud to believe that she had been particularly troubled by unresolved unconscious sexual feelings for her father and even an unconscious wish to bear his child. Freud considered it likely she would consequently have such feelings and wishes about Breuer. Early in her life she had established that way of relating to men in positions of authority. Further, he observed, she would tend to relate similarly to any man to whom she is attracted; that is, she would have sexual feelings and would also tend to repress them. Be-

cause such feelings were an unconscious replay of incestuous wishes, she would view them as forbidden. It is easy
to imagine that her unconscious ambivalences would cause
Bertha difficulty in her life. Indeed, the tendency to force
contemporary relationships into old patterns is likely to
cause difficulty for all of us. But as we will see, it can be an
invaluable ally to a therapist.

The Repetition Compulsion

The second discovery of Freud's that will help us in our
exploration of the clinical relationship is the one he called
the compulsion to repeat.[4] By this he meant that we have a
need to create for ourselves repeated replays of situations
and relationships that were particularly difficult or troubling in our early years. This was one of Freud's truly great
discoveries. We have all met people who go to remarkable
lengths to recreate situations that had bad endings.

Freud puts it like this:

> We have come across people all of whose human relationships have
> the same outcome: such as the benefactor who is abandoned in anger
> after a time by each of his *protégés*, however much they may otherwise
> differ from one another, and who thus seems doomed to taste all the
> bitterness of ingratitude; or the man whose friendships all end in
> betrayal by his friend; or the man who time after time in the course of
> his life raises someone else into a position of great private or public
> authority and then, after a certain interval, himself upsets that author-
> ity and replaces him by a new one; or, again, the lover each of whose
> love affairs passes through the same phases and reaches the same
> conclusion.[5]

The compulsion to repeat is a phenomenon that causes
dismay when we see it in our friends and despair when we
see it in ourselves. And it is a phenomenon with which we

are continually occupied in our work with clients. Like so much of human behavior, this seems paradoxical: Why go to such trouble to create a situation sure to cause one pain and frustration?

At first glance, it looks as though the person were trying over and over to put a happy ending on an earlier situation, one that had been anything but happy. But as we will see, it doesn't work that way. Should a replay turn out happily, the experience seems spoiled, and it's back to the drawing board to recreate the old unhappy situation once again. Freud's view was that the very painfulness of the original situation was fixating, driving one repeatedly to behave as though one were unconsciously trying to understand what had happened and why it had happened. We might thus expect Bertha to go to considerable lengths to put herself in situations reminiscent of her relationship with her father. Few of us would be surprised to learn that Bertha's father had actually been seductive toward her and that she had found in Breuer a man who was more than willing to play his part in a drama of seductive teasing.

We have noted that though a person in the grip of the repetition compulsion seems to be seeking a happy ending, such an interpretation is misguided. The situation with a happy ending would no longer be the *original* situation, which is defined by conflict, frustration, and guilt. So if Bertha ever had found a loving, attractive, slightly older man who returned her love and of whom all her friends and family approved, she would have been strongly motivated to lose interest in him and to resume the search for a desirable but forbidden man.

Since the repetition compulsion operates everywhere, it is no surprise that it turns up in the client's relationship with the therapist. And as we will see in the chapters ahead, that situation presents the therapist with valuable opportu-

24

nities. For one thing, it brings important parts of the client's life into the therapist's office, where they can be studied at close range. Further opportunities will become clear as we proceed.

Transference

According to Freud,[6] when people enter therapy, the way they see and respond to the therapist, and the reactions they set out to provoke are influenced by two tendencies: They will see the relationship in the light of their earliest ones, and they will try to engender replays of early difficult situations. To these perceptions, responses, and provocations, Freud gave the name *transference*, meaning that the client transfers onto the therapist the old patterns and repetitions.

As we will see in our discussion of Gill (Chapter 4), and particularly in the chapter on Kohut (Chapter 5), Freud's followers realized that transference could in some cases take a form other than the simple repetition of how the client had *experienced* the original relationship: it could also represent a replay of how the client had *wished* it were. So if I saw my father as aloof and disapproving I might see my analyst that way too, *or* I might see him or her as warm and loving, thus giving myself the "father" I always wanted. And I might switch back and forth between these.

The transference phenomenon is sufficiently strong to get itself expressed regardless of the gender of the therapist. While it is undoubtedly the case that at first a male therapist is more likely to draw a father transference and a female therapist a mother transference, eventually all the major relationships will get transferred onto the therapist, man or woman.

Two examples

One of my clients spent a good deal of the first year of her therapy raging at me. It didn't much matter what I did or didn't do; I was generally no good. Gradually she was able to tell me about being abandoned by her father at a very early age. It wasn't just that he had left her and her mother to fend for themselves; she had adored and completely trusted him. As I learned about this, I was able to accept her rage more easily and to understand why she needed to direct it toward me.

A male client often expressed concern about whether or not I liked him, admired him, preferred him to other clients. He had grown up in a cold home, with very constricted parents from a European culture that did not encourage the "coddling" of children. He was starved for validation. Kohut called this a "mirror transference," teaching that it represented the client's wish for affirmation never received.

Transference in everyday life

Freud has a featured place in the intellectual history of the twentieth century, not primarily because he pioneered a new approach to the treatment of emotional disturbance, but because he added significantly to our knowledge of ourselves. The theory of transference is a good example of his contribution. It doesn't apply only to clients and therapists; it applies to all of us in all our relationships. Everywhere we go, we are ceaselessly replaying some aspect or other of our early life. We can see it in our authority relations; we can see it in our love affairs; we can see it in our friendships; we can see it in our business dealings.

Becoming sensitive to the phenomena of transference doesn't only make us better clinicians; it also gives us a new appreciation for the astonishing design of our relationships. That design might be thought of as poetic or, more accurately perhaps, as musical.

The composers of the eighteenth and nineteenth centuries used a form they called the sonata. (The opening movements of Mozart's and Beethoven's symphonies are examples.) In the sonata all the themes that are going to appear are stated at the beginning. From there on, everything that occurs in the form is a variation, development, or replay of those themes. The listener's understanding and appreciation of those themes is continually increased. The power of that design is one of the reasons music of that period is apparently going to be played forever. One might think of one's first relationships as the themes of one's interpersonal life and all subsequent relationships as the development and recapitulation of those themes. We will see in the chapters ahead that this musical comparison gives us a productive way to view our clients.

Freud's way of understanding transference and of working with it evolved throughout his career. Following that evolution will help us grasp the concept.

Freud's early view of transference

Originally Freud saw the transference as being helpful if it consisted of positive feelings. Liking and wanting to please your therapist were seen as necessary motivations for the difficult journey. The only time positive feelings were *not* helpful, he noted, was when they had a strong erotic component that became so demanding and intractable that they interrupted or even wrecked the therapy.

A case in point is Bertha's powerful erotic transference to Breuer. Had the craft of psychoanalysis been sufficiently advanced at the time, Breuer might have been able to interpret the transference in its early stages and thus head off a sharp rupture of the therapy. The sad fact is that after the evening when Bertha told him she was pregnant, her treatment stopped, and they never saw each other again. But even if Breuer had seen what was coming and attempted to interpret it as transference, and even if his own countertransference — his own emotional involvement with his patient — had not been so strong, it's not certain he would have succeeded. In his paper, "Transference Love,"[7] Freud remarks that there are times when it is simply impossible to persuade a patient to give up the demand for the analyst's love and to accept the transference interpretation; then, according to Freud, the analysis is at an end.

The patient's inevitable *negative* feelings toward the therapist he saw as intermittent obstacles. The therapist's task was to "interpret the transference," that is, to help the patient understand the true (i.e., childhood) origins of these feelings, freeing the therapy from the burden of, say, suspicion or anger.

In one of his earliest published cases,[8] Freud writes of his patient Dora, who, to his surprise, abruptly terminated treatment. Only on reflection did Freud realize he had missed the signs that a severe negative transference was brewing and that his failure to have seen and interpreted it had been fatal to the analysis.

In Freud's early writings on this topic, transference interpretation was indicated only when the transference, whether erotic or negative, interfered with the patient's enthusiastic willingness to work with the therapist. Eventually he saw other reasons to work with the transference; we'll look at those in a moment.

At first, then, Freud believed that transference interpretation was not the real work of psychoanalysis and should be employed only when the transference got in the way of that real work. The "real work" of analysis consisted of reconstructing ancient dramas from the patient's free associations. They had to be reconstructed because they had been repressed, and could not have been consciously recalled even if the patient wanted to do so. And since they had been repressed, they operated without the patient's awareness and control and therefore had terrible destructive power.

Freud thought of himself as an archaeologist of the mind. He saw his work as reconstructing the hidden, unconscious story of the patient's life from clues and fragments, as a physical archaeologist attempts to reconstruct a civilization by carefully exhuming and assembling fragments of artifacts and bits of architecture. Reconstructing the ancient dramas meant making conscious their previously unconscious aspects. When these had been made conscious and "worked through" so that they could be "emotionally utilized" by the patient, they would no longer have the power to control the patient's life.

Working through and emotional utilization

Originally Freud had thought that merely discovering the unconscious dramas and explaining them to the patient would be sufficient for successful therapy. To his great disappointment, it was not. He discovered that "knowing" had many meanings. For example, patients could *know* intellectually that their guilt feelings were unjustified and *know* that their self-destructive patterns were generated by this guilt, and still, in an important sense, *not know* it. They could still hold the persistent old beliefs that pre-dated the analysis. These beliefs might be partly conscious; in spite of

29

the new knowledge, there might remain corners of consciousness in which the patients were not really *convinced* they did not deserve their guilt, and were not really *convinced* that they brought punishment down on their head in an attempt to alleviate that guilt. Though these perceptions might be partly conscious, they were likely to be predominantly unconscious: "If we communicate our knowledge to him, he does not receive it; and that makes very little change in it."[9] That is, unconsciously the patient clings to the old beliefs and the old blindnesses, and thus real change is unlikely. *Working through* was the name Freud gave to the process whereby these insights could be *emotionally utilized* and integrated into the personality, thus permitting the patient to give up his neurotic patterns.[10] This was Freud's way of dealing with the theme with which we began this book: Insight is not enough.

How the insights were to be worked through and integrated into the patient's personality became the main challenge of psychoanalysis. The importance of this cannot be overstated. Most of the subsequent history of psychotherapy, down to our own day, and most of the history of the clinical relationship, have consisted of attempts to solve that problem.

At first Freud thought that the way to permit the patient to work through insights was to have him encounter them over and over, in one context after another. That's why psychoanalysis took so long.

Early in my own psychoanalysis I learned how powerfully my life was influenced by guilt over fancied childhood sins. Then slowly, examining my life, I began learning about the multitude of ways that guilt manifested itself. I learned how it affected my work, how it shaped my relationships with women; I learned about its impact on my relations with my professors, as well as with supermarket clerks. I came to think that when psychoanalysis succeeded, it did so by boring a symptom to death. My analyst was applying Freud's early view of how insight becomes worked through and produces change in the patient. That view is still a part of psychoanalytic theory. But Freud was to add to it something new and important.

Working through in the transference

A significant moment in the history of psychoanalysis arrived when two lines of Freud's thought met and merged: his concern with the problem of emotional utilization of insights and his study of the clinical relationship. Why, Freud wondered, couldn't the insights be worked through in the relationship between the patient and the therapist? [11]

This, as you can see, marked an important change in the way he saw the clinical relationship, and indeed it marked a major change in the way any therapist had seen the relationship. He had taken two giant steps from the traditional view of doctor and patient. First, he had recognized that the nature of the relationship could facilitate or inhibit the analysis and that the analyst had some power to determine which of those effects it did indeed have. Second, he realized that an important part of the work of analysis could be done on the *subject* of the relationship itself.

What that meant was this: Previously the working through had been done by showing the patient how responses to early experiences shaped area after area of later life ("Can you see that you *expect* your teachers to be angry at you because of the old guilt you carry everywhere?"); now Freud was learning to add a new opportunity for understanding by showing the patient how the relationship to the *therapist* was shaped by those same responses. Psycho-analysis, itself, was an important event to the patient, and the analyst had now become an important person. Because of the transference, all the usual responses and all the typical distortions of the patient's life would be bound to show up in relation to the therapist. This would enable the therapist to demonstrate convincingly to the patient how early fantasies and impulses distort contemporary reality. Whatever interfered with the patient's life would show up clearly in the transference, so why not use the transference to help the patient see the distortions? Since the therapist had the data right there before them, wouldn't that make the learning all the more persuasive?

In *An Outline of Psychoanalysis* Freud says:

> It is the analyst's task constantly to tear the patient out of his . . . illusion [of the transference] and to show him again and again that what he takes to be new real life is a reflection of the past. . . . Careful handling of the transference . . . is as a rule richly rewarded. If we succeed, as we usually can, in enlightening the patient on the true nature of the phenomenon of transference, we shall have struck a powerful weapon out of the hand of his resistance and shall have converted dangers into gains. *For a patient never forgets again what he has experienced in the form of transference; it carries a greater force of conviction than anything he can acquire in other ways.* (Italics added)[12]

So somewhere between the professors and the checkout clerks I began learning how much I distorted my relationship with my analyst. I thought she was angry at me; I thought she neither liked nor approved of me; I thought she was disgusted by my fantasies. Sometimes she succeeded in getting me to see that I had no grounds for those ideas, that they were the products of that same unconscious guilt that so colored everything in my mind. And, indeed, learning about my guilt in relation to her did affect me more deeply than did learning about the professors and the checkout clerks.

We have seen, then, that Freud had first hoped that mere recall of the early impulses and relationships would be enough to effect change. When that hope was disappointed, he went on to hope that *repeated* recall would be more helpful. It *was* more helpful, but still not effective enough. Finally he hoped that a more convincing recall — recall in the transference — would so persuade the patient that all of his or her relationships were being distorted that change would simply have to follow. To his ever-growing disappointment, that seemed not to be enough either. A great deal was being learned about the mind, and some patients were undoubtedly being helped, but many were not.[13]

The theory of transference was a major discovery. The clinical relationship contains within it the whole story of the patient's problems, indeed the whole story of the patient's life. It is an astonishing microcosm. And it lays before the therapist a remarkable opportunity, not only for learning the secrets of the human mind, but for helping the patient as well. It was puzzling and painful to Freud that he had not found the way to extract the full potential from this opportunity.

As we follow the history of the post-Freudian work with transference, it will be helpful to keep two things in mind. First, Freud believed therapy was effected by *remembering*, by recalling the early material and realizing how it affected one's present life. Second, Freud saw transference primarily as *distortion* and believed that showing the patients those distortions could help them see the distortions throughout their lives.

Freud's work had made the greatest advances in the history of the field, but he had by no means solved all the problems. In subsequent chapters we will see how Gill and Kohut, two of the most imaginative among his followers, have learned to utilize the phenomenon of transference to develop a more effective clinical relationship.

For many years psychoanalysis was the only significant force in American clinical practice, until an American psychologist named Carl Rogers arrived on the scene. In the next chapter we'll look at his monumental contribution to our understanding of the relationship between therapist and client.

3

The Influence
of the Humanists

CARL ROGERS

I first read Carl Rogers' books in graduate school when I was immersed in the complex and fascinating world of academic psychology and the poetic vision of psychoanalysis. I found little to interest me in Rogers' writing. He was an American psychologist who believed the important parts of the mind were readily available to consciousness, he was cheerfully optimistic, and he seemed to have a predictable distaste for the dark aspects of European psychology. I thought he was mostly of historical interest.

Many years later, preparing a course, I set about rereading Rogers. I was utterly astonished. The simplicity of his view of the clinical relationship, which previously had seemed so naive to me, now seemed to have profound beauty and importance.

This book will end by proposing a therapy quite different from that which Rogers practiced and taught. But it seems to me that whatever view one holds of the human mind and however one chooses to conduct therapy, there is much to be learned by paying careful attention to Rogers' advice about the relationship between therapist and client.

Rogers' Great Influence

If *I* was not taken with Rogers' ideas when I first came across them, the same could not be said for the field of American clinical psychology. It would be an exaggeration to claim that the publication of Carl Rogers' *Counseling and Psychotherapy* in 1942[1] had the impact of say Freud's *The Interpretation of Dreams*, since Freud's books forever changed not only the practice of psychotherapy but also human beings' view of themselves. But excluding those by Freud, it is hard to name another set of books that has had an impact on clinical practice equal to Rogers'.

For a significant portion of the Western world's psycho-therapists he has legitimized the therapist's concern about the quality of the relationship between therapist and client; indeed, he has made that quality the therapist's paramount concern. Freud offered a radical new view of the mind, and drew from this view a set of remarkable inferences about how neurosis might be treated. The key word was *treated*. As we have seen, Freud was a physician, and he saw neurosis as an illness to be cured. Rogers' background was different. He was not a physician, and he did not view emotional difficulties as an indication of an illness to be cured. He called the people with whom he worked, "clients," rather than "patients." He had at one time planned on being a minister, and though he abandoned that career, his religious predilection can be seen in his view of psychology. He believed that human beings needed to be loved, and when their need was inadequately met, the result was confusion and pain. If someone could give the suffering person a significant experience of the love so sorely missing, the confusion and pain would go away by itself.

A Therapy of Love

Rogers seldom said he was offering a therapy of love, and his way of helping people change was certainly different from the mushy sentimentality that characterizes some "new age" therapists. But I think it will help our understanding of his monumental contribution to our field to realize that he was indeed introducing into it the variable of love.

By "love," Rogers meant that which the Greeks named *agape*. Greek philosophy distinguished between two kinds of love, *eros* and *agape*. *Eros* is characterized by the desire for something that will fulfill the *lover*. It includes the wish to possess the beloved object or person. *Agape*, on the other hand, is characterized by the desire to fulfill the *beloved*. It demands nothing in return and wants only the growth and fulfillment of the loved one. *Agape*, is a strengthening love, a love that, by definition, does not burden or obligate the loved one.

Rogers spent 40 years developing his view of therapy. And perhaps it would not be far off the mark to view his whole 40 years' work as an attempt to shape an answer to a single question: What would a therapist do to convey to a client that at last he or she is loved?

To answer that question, Rogers and his student spent countless hours studying the process of psychotherapy. He was the first to make audio recordings of sessions and permit them to be studied and analyzed. He believed that therapy could be studied scientifically and continually improved by that research.[2]

Although Rogers developed a well-articulated theory of personality, he came to believe that it didn't matter what theory of personality you held. If the therapist successfully communicated the experience of *agape*, the client would change in the desired direction. Not only didn't the theory matter, neither did the technique. You could practice the nondirective, client-centered reflection that Rogers had developed in earlier years, or you could interpret free-associations in the classic psychoanalytic manner, do Gestalt exercises, or analyze the transference. It didn't matter. Whatever suited the theory and style of the therapist was fine as long as *agape* was successfully communicated.[3]

What *did* matter, and it mattered considerably, was how *agape* was communicated. Rogers and his students had studied the problem assiduously for many years, and Rogers believed he knew what worked and what didn't. What he thought worked was a therapy that communicated to the client *genuineness, empathy*, and *unconditional positive regard*. Let's look at each of those concepts in detail.

Genuineness

Therapists must be *genuine* or, as Rogers sometimes said, "congruent." That means they must have ongoing access to their own internal process, their own feelings, their own attitudes, and their own moods. Rogers believed that therapists who were not receptive to the awareness of their own flow of feeling and thought would be unlikely to help clients become aware of theirs. Undoubtedly there are therapists who choose this profession because they imagine that focusing on the client's internal process is a good way to avoid the pain and anxiety of looking at their own. Rogers teaches that this is a recipe for disaster. Becoming a therapist means taking on an awesome responsibility for facing oneself. Certainly the early psychoanalysts had understood this, though this understanding was sometimes only a peripheral aspect of the analysts' orientation, and too often it disappeared altogether. Rogers insisted on its being central.

If genuineness means being aware of one's thoughts and feelings, it also means that therapists must do nothing to conceal this inner process from the client. They must not be defensive, but rather must be *transparent*. It is important to note that this concept implies nothing at all about what therapists are to say or do. It only suggests that they are to present themselves transparently, with nothing concealed. They may do this silently with their inner qualities revealed in their eyes, face, and posture. Or they may choose at certain times to tell the client what they are feeling.

Rogers confesses he is puzzled by just how much therapists ought actually to *say* to the client about their feelings or attitudes. He is clear that genuineness does *not* mean blurting out every passing feeling. He is not, therefore, suggesting a form of "encounter" therapy in which the therapist shares every feeling with the client. He thinks that genuineness perhaps means expressing a feeling only when it has persisted and when it seems to be interfering with the therapist's ability to be fully present for the client. And then the feeling is to be presented carefully, with warmth, empathy, and full respect for the client. Let me quote here one of Rogers' examples:

> But is it always helpful to be genuine? What about negative feelings? What about the times when the counselor's real feeling toward the client is one of annoyance or boredom or dislike? My tentative answer is that even with such feelings as these, which we all have from time to time, it is preferable for the counselor to be real than to put up a facade of interest and concern and liking, which he does not feel.
> But it is not a simple thing to achieve such reality. Being real involves the difficult task of being acquainted with the flow of expe-

39

riencing going on within oneself, a flow marked especially by complexity and continuous change. So if I sense that I am feeling bored by my contacts with this [client], and this feeling persists, I think I owe it to him and to our relationship to share this feeling with him. But here again I will want to be constantly in touch with what is going on in me. I will recognize that it is *my* feeling of being bored which I am expressing, and not some supposed fact about him as a boring person. If I voice it as *my own* reaction, it has the potentiality of leading to a deeper relationship. But this feeling exists in the context of a complex and changing flow, and this needs to be communicated too. I would like to share with him my distress at feeling bored, and the discomfort I feel in expressing this aspect of me. As I share these attitudes I find that my feeling of boredom arises from my sense of remoteness from him, and that I would like to be more in touch with him. And even as I try to express these feelings, they change. I am certainly *not* bored as I try to communicate myself to him in this way, and I am far from bored as I wait with eagerness and perhaps a bit of apprehension for his response. I also feel a new sensitivity to him, now that I have shared this feeling which has been a barrier between us. So I am very much more able to hear the surprise or perhaps the hurt in his voice as he now finds *him*self speaking more genuinely because I have dared to be real with him. I have let myself be a person — real, imperfect — in my relationship with him.[4]

Rogers cautions therapists against using this sort of advice as a license to work out their own issues on the client's time, and he reminds his readers that often the appropriate person with whom to share their feelings is a supervisor or colleague, not the client.

In spite of the amount of time and energy Rogers devoted to writing about genuineness (he wrote about it in article after article), he seemed to find this attribute hard to describe and to illustrate. But it seems clear that intuitively he knew what he meant. At some level we all recognize when we are face to face with a person who is being genuine with us and when we are with someone who is putting on a polite or professional facade. With the former we feel trust and willingness to expose ourselves. It is this quality Rogers was trying to describe.

Rogers thought genuineness the most important attribute of all.

Empathy

The second condition essential to successful therapy is *empathy*. The dictionary meaning of *empathy* is the imaginative entering of another's subjective experience. Rogers is talking about the importance of the therapist's continually trying to understand the client's experience *from the client's point of view*. To Rogers, empathy is not merely cognitive; it also includes an emotional, experiential component. It means attempting to experience the client's world the way the client experiences it, but experiencing it without getting lost in it, without ever losing the "as if" quality.

Whether the client is experiencing fear or uncertainty, loneliness or anger, admiration or disappointment toward the therapist, empathic therapists allows themselves to experience what the client is experiencing and do their best to communicate that understanding and experience to the client:

> "It must be very frightening to be so uncertain about your job security. And I also imagine you must be pretty angry at your boss."

> "I think I see what you're saying. In some ways you like coming here and talking to me, but you're not sure it's really doing very much for you."

> "My goodness, you really love her, don't you?"

Rogers puts it like this:

> To sense [the client's] confusion or his timidity or his anger or his feeling of being treated unfairly as if it were your own, yet without your own uncertainty or fear or anger or suspicion getting bound up in it, this is the condition I am endeavoring to describe. When the client's world is clear to the counselor and she can move about in it freely, then she can both communicate her understanding of what is vaguely known to the client, and she can also voice meanings in the client's experience of which the client is scarcely aware.[5]

Two of Rogers' students, C. B. Truax and R. R. Carkhuff, describe the empathic therapist.[6] Here is a somewhat simplified summary:

Empathic Therapists:

Have a manner and tone that indicate they take this relationship seriously.

Are aware of what the client is feeling now.

Have a capacity to *communicate this understanding* in a language attuned to those current feelings.

Make their comments in a way that *fits* with the client's mood and content. These comments indicate sensitive understanding of feelings the client has actually expressed and also serve to clarify and expand the client's awareness of feelings and experiences, including those of which the client is only partly aware.

Are able to stay in tune with the client's shifting emotional content so that they can correct themselves when they discover that their understanding and their comments have been off-target. They are sensitive to their mistakes and do not cling to them, but easily and nonde-fensively change their response in midstream.

Continually give the client the message, "I am with you."

Unfortunately this sort of understanding is rare in our ordinary lives. It doesn't often happen that parent or teacher, friend or lover really tries to grasp what a given experience is like for us or that we try to grasp what one is like for them. In everyday life the understanding we tend to give and receive is some form of "I understand what makes you act that way" or "I understand what's wrong with you." Traditionally much of clinical understanding has been similar to this:

"I think you're actually very angry at women."

"Perhaps you're focusing so much on my inadequacies to avoid looking at your feelings about this matter."

To Rogers this isn't understanding at all; it is evaluation and analysis. It is viewing other people's lives in our terms, not in theirs.

The therapeutic value of *empathic* understanding seems clear: When I really *get* it that my therapist is trying to see my world the way I see it, I feel encouraged to clarify and therefore increase my understanding of myself. This em-pathy teaches me to be empathic with myself, to try gently to grasp my experience in the accepting way my therapist grasps it. And like all *agape*, another's empathy has a crucial effect on my self-esteem. If my therapist thinks it worth the time and effort to try to understand my experience, *I* must be worth the time and effort.

Unconditional positive regard

The third necessary quality of the effective therapist is *unconditional positive regard*. Rogers takes the position that if I'm not on your side, *really* on your side, I have no business being in a therapy office with you. His model for this attribute is the loving parent who "prizes" the child. Such a parent has strong positive feelings for the child, feelings that are not possessive and do not demand that the child be a certain way. The parent gives the message that, even though from time to time the child is likely to evoke annoyance, anger, disapproval, or disgust, the child is basically, essentially, loved and lovable, no matter what. Similarly, a client may (and almost certainly will) reveal feelings and behaviors that clash with the therapist's values or aesthetics. Successful therapy depends on the therapist's being able at such times to keep in view that clients are worthwhile human beings struggling gamely to find their way back to their birthright of growth and self-development, and as such, should be *prized*.

It is important in Rogers' view that this feeling be neither paternalistic nor sentimental and that it give the client a great deal of room to be a separate and independent person.

If I go to a surgeon for a medical problem, the surgeon may not like me or even have any respect for me. I may find the situation a bit unpleasant, but if the surgeon is skilled and responsible, I will probably come out about as well as if I had been prized. Rogers taught that holding medicine as an analogue for psychotherapy has led to serious difficulties in the practice of therapy and the training of therapists. We are not *doing* therapy the way the surgeon does surgery; we *are* the therapy, and without a substantial amount of unconditional positive regard, we will not be successful.

Few of us had parents capable of that kind unconditional prizing. Many of us learned that we were loved only when we did something or revealed some feeling that pleased our parents. It might be something convenient for them, or nonthreatening to them, or something they could be proud of. Many of our feelings, wishes, and impulses did not fit the category of "pleasing to our parents." We quickly learned that those feelings and impulses were unlovable, and it was a short step to come to believe they were *bad*. It is easy to understand how we then lost touch with our deepest nature:

If I have been taught that to be lovable I must harbor only good feelings and good impulses,

And if I have become convinced that my true self is full of bad feelings and bad impulses,

Then I will set about trying to disavow the parts of me about which I have such gloomy suspicions.

If a goal of the therapist is to make it safe for clients to explore their deepest nature, we can see why Rogers thought that unconditional positive regard was essential.

The Three Attributes as Continua

Genuineness, empathy, and unconditional positive regard, these, then, are the three attributes that Rogers thought necessary to a successful clinical relationship. I'm sure it has occurred to you that if any of us could always be fully genuine, empathic, and warmly accepting, we would be in a state of Nirvana or in heaven and not available to earthly clients. It had occurred to Rogers, too. He did not think that any mortal would ever be perfect in any of the three. Rather, he saw each of these attributes as a continuum and believed that the art of becoming a therapist consisted *entirely* in developing one's capacity to move further and further along each of those three continua. The farther along one was, the better therapist one would be.

The Implication's of Rogers' Theory

The implications of this point of view are extraordinarily radical. Note the word "entirely" in the above paragraph. One implication of Rogers' views is that no special intellectual or professional knowledge is required of therapists or will do them the slightest good. Studying theories and techniques, however interesting they may be, are not of value to the therapist.[7] Training could be helpful, in fact very helpful, but that training would not consist of the acquisition of knowledge. It would be experiential training, the sort of training that would help therapists increase their self-awareness so that they might become more genuine everywhere in their lives, including with their clients. It would be a training that would increase their sensitivity to other people everywhere in their lives, so that they might be more empathic with clients. And it would be a training that would enable them to come to terms with their buried prejudices and resentments so that they might be free to prize their clients.

As I have said, Rogers did not consider himself an "encounter" therapist; he didn't see it as appropriate to share every passing feeling with the client. Yet in the early 1960s he began spending more and more time leading encounter groups and sensitivity-training groups. He saw these groups as offering the sort of training that developed the attributes he thought essential to a therapist. He greatly regretted that almost nowhere was such sensitivity enhancement a part of the formal training of therapists.[8]

Another radical implication of Rogers' viewpoint is that there is no therapeutic value in diagnosis.[9] That is, having a category into which the client may be fitted adds nothing to the therapist's effectiveness. It doesn't make any difference whether someone thinks your client is borderline or narcissistic or schizophrenic or mildly depressed. If you can be genuine, if you can communicate that you are managing to grasp your client's experience, and if you can let them know of your unshakable regard for their worth as human beings — if you can do all that to a significant degree, then the clients will grow and change, whatever label might be applied to them. (Rogers did come to believe that clients not motivated to change were hard to work with and unlikely to change very much. He found that many people diagnosed as schizophrenic were unmotivated — as were a lot of people not so diagnosed.)

Rogers' idea about the components of successful therapy clearly implies a certain philosophical attitude. Rogers believed the purpose of life is "to be that which one truly is."[10] Our clients are in trouble because they have been successfully taught that it is *not acceptable* to be what they truly are. Thus Rogers asks therapists to do their best to *listen* as carefully as possible in order to find out who the client truly is. As the therapist carefully attends, the client gradually learns that it is all right to be whomever he or she truly is, and since Rogers believes that being one's true self is the purpose of life, it is easy to see why he thinks self-acceptance is the most valuable thing a therapist can give a client.

Rogers says that in order to find his work useful, a therapist probably ought to hold a philosophical position similar to his own.[11] One who does not, is likely to try to guide clients into being what *the therapist* thinks they ought to be. Rogers believes that some therapists' attitudes are simply not congenial with the point of view he offers. Some examples of those incompatible attitudes:

People are neither valuable nor unvaluable; they are simply interesting to try to figure out.

They may not even be particularly interesting, but they furnish material for books and articles, which is to say for ideas, and ideas certainly *are* interesting.

The therapist soon learns all there is of interest to learn about the client. The rest of the work consists of getting the client to learn it.

The therapist's theory handles all the data. When enough knowledge has been gathered, the client will fit the theory.

Clients can't be trusted to find their own way. If left to their own devices, they will resist, defend, and do whatever they can to impede change and growth. The therapist's job is to protect the client against those self-destructive tendencies.

That is, the therapist knows better than the clients what is good for him and tries to figure out a way to influence them for their own good.

But if the therapist believes in the essential worth of the individual, if the context in which the therapist works is one of great respect for the person and the person's potentialities, then, Rogers thought, that therapist would find the attributes of genuineness, empathy, and warm acceptance congenial, natural, and altogether understandable.

Concluding Remarks

In 1961 Rogers wrote a description of what he thought therapy was like at its best. It seems like a good way to close this chapter:

> If the therapy were optimal, intensive as well as extensive, then it would mean that the therapist has been able to enter into an intensely personal and subjective relationship with the client—relating not as a scientist to an object of study, not as a physician expecting to diagnose and cure, but as a person to a person. It would mean that the therapist feels this client to be a person of unconditional self-worth: of value no matter what his condition, his behavior, or his feelings. It would mean that the therapist is genuine, hiding behind no defensive façade, but meeting the client with the feelings which organically he is experiencing. It would mean that the therapist is able to let himself go in understanding this client; that no inner barriers keep him from sensing what it feels like to be the client at each moment of the relationship; and that he can convey something of his empathic understanding to the client. It means that the therapist has been comfortable in entering this relationship fully, without knowing cognitively where it will lead, satisfied with providing a climate which will permit the client the utmost freedom to become himself.
>
> For the client, the optimal therapy would mean an exploration of increasingly strange and unknown and dangerous feelings in himself, the exploration proving possible only because he is gradually realizing that he is accepted unconditionally. Thus be becomes acquainted with elements of his experience which have in the past been denied to awareness as too threatening, too damaging to the structure of the self. He finds himself experiencing these feelings fully, completely, in the relationship, so that for the moment he *is* his fear, or his anger, or

his tenderness, or his strength. And as he lives these widely varied feelings, in all their degrees of intensity, he discovers that he has experienced *himself*, that he *is* all these feelings. He finds his behavior changing in constructive fashion in accordance with his newly experienced self. He approaches the realization that he no longer needs to fear what experience may hold, but can welcome it freely as a part of his changing and developing self." [12]

4

A Re-experiencing Therapy

MERTON GILL

M erton Gill, M.D., is a long-time member of the psychoanalytic establishment and one of its most eminent. Few members of the psychoanalytic community have thought as deeply or written as influentially about the clinical relationship as Merton Gill.[1]

Though Gill is a psychoanalyst, he is quite explicit in saying that his views on the clinical relationship do not pertain merely to psychoanalysis, but to all forms of psychodynamic therapy, including that which occurs once or twice a week.[2]

What About Therapy Is Therapeutic?

Remembering . . .?

Perhaps the best way to understand Gill's contribution to our topic is to wonder for a moment what about therapy is therapeutic. To Freud, therapy comes about from the patient's *remembering* thoughts and feelings long repressed. To understand that, it might be helpful to review a few basic elements of Freud's theory of psychopathology.

To Freud, the human is the species that represses itself. The fate of humans is to be caught in intense, persistent conflict. Regardless of what the socializing community does or doesn't do, the conflicts arise from human nature itself. Mental life is driven by powerful instincts; these instincts clash with each other, and they clash with the reality constraints of the outside world.[3-5] And before the child is very old, he or she has a sizable collection of fears, something else for the instincts to clash with. Thus conflict is everywhere. When one of these conflicts becomes sufficiently intense, it becomes too painful to keep in awareness, and so it is repressed; that is, it is relegated to the realm of unconsciousness. This constitutes a successful short-term solution to the problem of painful awareness, and in modest doses it's an adaptive long-term solution as well. Our mental life would be unacceptably chaotic without a moderate amount of repression. *Excessive* repression, on the other hand, causes serious long-term consequences:

1. It takes a significant amount of psychic energy to keep an impulse in repression. That energy is not available for living one's life.

2. Repressed material is by definition unconscious and therefore not under the control of the conscious, rational faculties; that is, it's not under the control of that part of the mind Freud called the *ego*. Thus it may cause all sorts of trouble. We saw several instances of this kind of trouble in Chapter 2, in our examination of the repetition compulsion.

3. Repressed material acts as a magnet, drawing other impulses into the unconscious. If I have passionate im-

pulses toward my mother, it is healthy and adaptive for me to repress them. But if that area of repression spreads to include passionate impulses toward all women, my life will be difficult indeed.

Freud believed that it was excessive repression that created problems for his patients. Their lives were being pushed around by inner forces of which they were unaware and they therefore could not control. As we saw in Chapter 2, Freud hoped that if he could make the repressed material conscious, and if that new consciousness could somehow be emotionally utilized, that is, made an effective part of the patient's awareness, the problems would be meliorated. In other words, he wanted his patients to *remember* and to remember with conviction.[6]

Imagine a man who suffers from an inability to experience both passionate and tender feelings toward the same woman. He might feel passionate toward one sort of woman and tender toward another, but he can't feel both toward any one woman. Freud would attribute this incapacity to the man's having repressed early impulses and memories relating to conflicting feelings of desire and fear—desire for his mother and fear of punishment for those desires. Thus women toward whom he feels tender are categorized as being "like mother." Passionate feelings toward such women are unconsciously seen as incestuous and are forbidden. Freud believed that once the memory of those feelings and the events associated with them could be recaptured and once those memories could be worked through, the problem would be significantly lessened. This is *remembering* therapy.

Freud set himself two goals when working with a patient. One was to ease the patient's neurotic suffering. The other goal was to use the information gleaned from the patient to help construct a theory of the mind. To the end of his life he believed that these two tasks were not only compatible, but were the same. That is, he believed that the truth would make his patients free. If he could unearth the secrets of this patient's unconscious, if he could thoroughly convince the patient that his hidden story was the root of his suffering, then the patient's expanded knowledge would perform the therapeutic transformation. And Freud believed that, as he learned this patient's hidden story, he would be simultaneously learning the hidden story of humankind. Beneath the facade of human consciousness lay an amazing puzzle, a captivating mystery. And the patient's buried story contained the ingredients of the solution.

Ever since, psychoanalysis has attracted practitioners who are puzzle solvers, therapists who want to get to the bottom of the mystery and who share Freud's belief that this fascination with the puzzles of psychic life is in the patient's best interest.

Gill represents a growing number of modern psychoanalysts who, though they find a great deal of Freud's work indispensable, no longer believe that uncovering the hidden story is enough to liberate the client. For generations now, with client after client, psychoanalysts have succeeded in unearthing the unconscious fantasies that give rise to symptoms and have succeeded in convincingly communicating this analysis to clients, but in a discouraging number of cases the symptoms remain. The client has *remembered* the old impulses and the old fears. But remembering has not been enough.

. . . Or Re-experiencing?

Gill and like-minded colleagues accept Freud's theory of psychopathology, and although they believe that remembering is necessary to effect significant change in therapy, they find that it is not sufficient. Actually, Freud himself had doubts about whether remembering was sufficient. Though his published clinical work indicates his unflagging commitment to the recapturing of lost memories, there are places in his theoretical writings where can be found the basis for re-experiencing therapy. One of many examples:

> . . . the whole of the patient's illness . . . is concentrated on a single point—his relation to the doctor. . . . When the transference has risen to this significance, work upon the patient's memories retreats far into the background. Thereafter it is not incorrect to say that we are no longer concerned with the patient's earlier illness but with a newly created and transformed neurosis which has taken the former's place.[7]

If remembering is not enough, what is missing is *re-experiencing*. Gill believes that, because the client's difficulties were acquired experientially, they must be transformed experientially. They cannot be reasoned away. While it is necessary for clients eventually to understand the roots of their difficulties, that understanding cannot be delivered as an explanation. It must emerge from the clients' re-experiencing certain aspects of their past. And this re-experiencing must occur within the therapeutic relationship. Gill says:

> The transference is primarily a result of the patient's efforts to realize his wishes, and the therapeutic gain result primarily from re-experiencing these wishes in the transference, realizing that they are significantly determined by something preexisting within the patient, and experiencing something new in examining them together with the analyst—the one to whom the wishes are now directed.[8]

Thus a re-experiencing therapist believes that the client must have an opportunity to relive emotionally the impulses, the anxieties, and the conflicts of his past and to relive them under certain specified conditions. How that might be brought about is the topic of this chapter.

Conditions for Therapeutic Re-experiencing

According to Gill, for re-experiencing to be therapeutic, the impulses and feelings must be experienced under the following conditions:

1. They must be experienced in the presence of the person toward whom they are now directed.

2. The re-experienced feelings must be *expressed* toward the person toward whom they are now directed. It is not enough for the client merely to experience the feelings silently.

It seems so far that it should be therapeutic for the old feelings to be re-experienced toward *anyone* as long as they are expressed to that person. That leads to the next condition:

3. The new object of the old feelings, the person toward whom they are now directed, must be willing, even determined, to discuss the client's feelings and impulses with interest, objectivity, and without defensiveness. According to Gill, this is absolutely essential to the therapeutic process. Given the low probability of encountering such a response in our ordinary lives, we begin to see why Gill views the opportunity of the therapeutic situation as unique.

4. The client must be helped to learn the ancient and deep source of the re-experienced impulses. Thus, re-

membering and re-experiencing become organically blended.

So Freud's troubled patient who cannot combine love and desire will sooner or later find himself experiencing toward the therapist (irrespective of whether the therapist is a man or woman) impulses he considers forbidden. As we saw in our chapter on Freud, the repetition compulsion demands this.

If the therapist:

Helps the client get in touch with these feelings,

Makes it safe for the client to express them,

Discusses these feelings with the client in a nonjudgmental, nondefensive, interested fashion,

And eventually, when the therapy has progressed far enough, helps the client learn the ancient roots of these feelings,

then Gill's conditions for therapeutic re-experiencing have been met.

It is worth noting here that it is not only modern psychoanalysts who have come to believe that figuring out the cause of the symptom is not enough. Most schools of therapy hold some version of this belief; so do many psychologists who are not therapists. Psychologists who study the laws of learning think about it this way: In the learning laboratory the easiest way to get an animal or a person to *unlearn* an old response is to recreate the situation in which that response was originally learned. In fact, it can be hard to get someone to unlearn a response if you *don't* recreate the old situation. Freud's patient has learned the response of sexual inhibition to the stimulus of a "motherlike" woman. The learning psychologist would see this patient as needing to unlearn that response and learn a new one — one that better suits present needs. The psychologist would doubt that it would do much good merely to explain to the patient how the old response was acquired. Therapists of many persuasions would agree (though most would be unlikely to express it in just that language or to arrive at the learning psychologist's solution.) These therapists commonly believe that the old pain or the old impulse must be re-experienced in therapy; each school has its own way of trying to bring this about. To many modern psychoanalysts, including Gill, the optimal place for the re-experiencing is the relationship with the therapist.

A New Importance Seen in Transference

The emphasis on re-experiencing represents an important change in the psychoanalytic view of transference. To Freud, the value of transference lay in its power to help the patient remember and remember with conviction. To Gill, the value of transference lies in providing the client a chance to experience once more the old impulses. The response *originally* encountered by expression of those impulses generated the pain and confusion that eventually brought the client to the therapist. As they are re-experienced in the transference, now directed at the person of the therapist, they will receive a significantly different response. To Gill, this is the main therapeutic opportunity provided by the phenomenon of transference.

This view of therapy implies that it is to clients' advantage to be more and more in touch with their experience of the therapist and of the relationship. This includes their

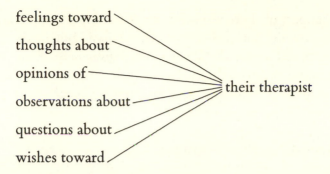

and importantly, the feelings, thoughts, opinions, observations, questions, and wishes that clients believe their therapist has about them.

The Inevitability of Resistance

It is understandably frightening for the client to contemplate experiencing, let alone expressing, any but the mildest and safest feelings toward the therapist. It is not easy to tell *anyone* our feelings, impressions, or fantasies about him or her. How much harder it is when we are depending on that person for significant help. And when we recall that this developing relationship with the therapist carries with it more and more unconscious reminders of our earliest and most difficult times, we can understand how determinedly the client is likely to resist all aspects of transference — experiencing it, revealing it, learning its roots.

The most important and delicate job facing the therapist is to help the client through this resistance, so that the client's awareness of thoughts and feelings about the therapist, however subtle and however disguised, may continually increase. Later we will see how Gill helps clients learn which of these thoughts and feelings are *transference*, that is, what part of those responses are determined not merely by the present, but also by the client's past. But in the early phases of therapy all he is trying to do is help clients learn just how occupied they are with their relationship with the therapist. We can see how important this step is to a re-experiencing therapist.[9]

Decoding the Transference

To help clients become aware of their relationship with the therapist, the therapist must first be sensitive to the fact that allusions to the therapeutic situation are likely to be *encoded*, often as references to other situations. Second, from moment to moment, the therapist must be sensitive to what is going on in the therapeutic situation in order to have some idea what stimuli the client is responding to. If the client begins talking about feeling criticized at the job, the therapist will scan recent events in the therapy to see whether any of them might have made the client feel criticized. If that scan turns up a possibility, the therapist sets out to decode, as tactfully and respectfully as possible, the client's statement about the situation.

Gill places great emphasis on tact and respect, reminding us that clients say what they mean, and what they say is of great importance to them. Gill hopes that a therapist would not say, "What you mean is that you feel criticized by me" or "What you are really saying is that you feel criticized by me." The client neither said nor meant that. Rather, a sensitive therapist might say, "I can understand that feeling criticized at work is very disturbing to you. And I wonder if an additional meaning of what you say is that in our last session you felt criticized by me."[10]

To the re-experiencing school of psychoanalysts, the relationship is central; it is what makes the re-experiencing possible. As the therapist encourages awareness of the client's experience of the relationship, clients becomes more aware of their shifting and developing attitudes toward the therapist. In addition, that relationship assumes greater and greater importance to them. Thus the relationship becomes the microcosm of their lives — their confusions, ways of relating, longings and disappointments, their hopes and frustrations. During the therapeutic hour, after all, all other relationships are abstract, are at a distance. Only the therapeutic relationship is right there in the room and thus available to exploration with a unique depth, immediacy, and power.

This means that although Gill finds value in discussing a client's life outside the therapeutic situation, he assigns to such discussion a somewhat lower priority than he does to life within the situation. And that raises this question: Is it true that so much of what the client says really pertains to the therapist? Gill would replace that question with this one: Whether or not it's *true*, is it *useful* to operate on that assumption? And Gill's experience leads him to answer yes to that question.

Since encouraging awareness of the relationship is so important in Gill's system, let's look at some examples:

1. Often the transference is coded as being about a relationship with another person: "I'm starting to trust my lover a bit more, I think." The therapist will acknowledge that this is an important change in the client's life and give the topic as much time and attention as seems useful. Later, at an appropriate time, the therapist will look for a graceful opportunity to add: I'm aware that we had a good session last week. I wonder if an additional meaning of what you say about your lover is that you're starting to have more trust in me."

Gill gives the example of a client who expresses worry about losing his housekeeper. The therapist suggests the client may also be worried about an impending interruption in the therapy caused by the therapist's vacation.

Another example of Gill's concerns a client complaining about his wife's making unreasonable demands on him. The therapist realizes that he has recently been involved in negotiating an appointment time with the client and wonders aloud if the client has found *him* demanding and unreasonable.[11]

2. Sometimes the transference is coded as being about another situation: "I went to a party last night, and the atmosphere was so heavy and depressing." The therapist will convey understanding of how that must have felt, and then, when it seems feasible, will say, "Your talking about the party last night raises another question. We've been having difficult sessions lately, and I wonder if you're also finding the atmosphere in here a bit heavy as well."

3. The transference may also be coded as an expression of concern about how another person feels about the client: "I really want to know how my boss feels about me. I can't stand this uncertainty." The therapist will acknowledge how difficult this must be and, after the discussion about the boss, might say, "Is it possible that you also have some questions about how I feel about you?"

A common sequence is an initial glancing reference to the therapy situation followed by a description of a relationship or situation outside the therapy.[12] The client says:

"That was a good session last week. (*pause*) I'm starting to trust my lover a bit more, I think."

"I really didn't want to come in today. (*pause*) I went to a party last night, and the atmosphere was so heavy and depressing."

"I was thinking this week that I talk a lot more in here than you do. (*pause*) I really want to know how my boss feels about me. I can't stand this uncertainty."

In these instances the therapist's job is made easier, because the plausibility of the interpretation is enhanced by the client's tangential reference to the transference.

Liberating the Therapist's Warmth and Spontaneity

The classic view of psychoanalysis held that all of the cues of the analytic environment should be as neutral as the analyst. There should be nothing in the physical environment to give definite messages to the client about the person who furnished and who inhabits this office. The analyst should be silent, noncommittal, and nonresponsive. Above all, there should be no clue as to the personality or the values of the analyst. As we have seen, all of this was to provide a blank screen onto which clients could project their transferences, uncontaminated by reality.

To Gill, this is not neutrality at all. Someone who says neither hello nor good-bye, who doesn't answer questions, who remains silent under severe provocation, is hardly neutral. When one feels cold and lonely with such a person, Gill says, it shouldn't be assumed that these feelings come from one's childhood. Who *wouldn't* feel cold and lonely in the face of that kind of treatment?

63

This raises an important issue. Psychoanalysts regularly observe that the analytic situation produces a considerable amount of regressed transference material: Clients experience themselves as very young and as occupied with primitive needs. A client may, for instance, feel like a starving baby who wants to beg the analyst for nurturance. At such times it is commonly assumed that the analysis has revealed something deep and important about the client's history, that is, that long ago the client actually felt that way. Undoubtedly that is often the case. But it seems likely that sometimes this material is not revealing the client's history at all but is actually being created by the excessively cold ambience the analyst has created in pursuit of neutrality.[13]

Providing the client with a "blank screen" is manifestly impossible; the situation is going to be rife with clues whatever I do as a therapist, so I might as well permit myself a good deal of spontaneity. This will not only create a more therapeutic atmosphere, but will also liberate my own creativity: It seems likely that if I am putting stringent restrictions on my behavior, my cognitive, imaginative, and expressive capacities are going to be correspondingly restricted. Thus some degree of therapist's spontaneity seems very much in the client's interest.

Such freedom carries with it responsibility: the responsibility for therapists to pay close attention to all the elements of the situation, including the things they do and the ways in which they do them. The client's reactions will be strongly influenced by two things: (1) what is actually happening in therapy and (2) the expectations, needs, and attitude brought by the client into the situation. It is important to recognize that the client's responses are determined *by what the therapist does*, as well as by the forces of transference.

In thus seeing therapy as an *interpersonal* situation, Gill differs from the classical analysts who tried hard to be nonpersons, who believed they had successfully created a blank screen, and who perhaps underestimated how much what they did and didn't do contributed to the client's experience. Just as a dream, Gill says, uses the events of the preceding day as opportunities to explore deep content, so the client will use elements from the actual therapeutic situation as the material from which the transference phenomena are elaborated. Gill says, "[It is an error to believe that therapy] develops in a social vacuum. The therapist may deny that he is reacting to the patient, but it is impossible for him to avoid such reaction. . . . The therapist who does not recognize the inevitably social nature of the therapeutic situation is in the grip of the companion illusion to the illusion of himself as a blank screen. . . . It is the illusion that the patient is naive."[14]

Let's look at a couple of examples:

1. The client is particularly witty and the therapist indulges in hearty laughter. It's not done for any technical reason, but just because the therapist was permitting herself some spontaneity. As she laughs, she recognizes the possibility that this might have some meaning to the client, and she makes a mental note of it. Later in the session the client speaks of a professor who clowns around in class so much that little is learned.

Therapist: I can imagine that would be distressing. I also wonder if it's significant that you bring it up now. Perhaps you have some feeling that if I'm having too good a time in here, I'm not working as well as I might.

2. The client, although not a particularly "political" type, spends some minutes criticizing liberals who would give everything away to the poor. The therapist, who considers himself a liberal, is puzzled by what seems unusual and out of context and wonders how this might possibly be about him. Suddenly he looks at his overcoat hanging on a coat rack and realizes that a political button on the lapel is in plain sight from the office. He now has an opening for investigating how the material relates to him.

Gill has some advice that would apply to this situation in the event that the therapist has not seen the button. Were the therapist sufficiently puzzled by the political material, it would seem to Gill altogether appropriate to say, "You know, I keep wondering if an additional meaning of what you are saying relates to me. Do you have some thoughts about my politics?" The client might then mention the button or merely say that he imagines most psychotherapists are liberals.

To repeat: There's no way, Gill says, to keep reality stimuli out of the situation. Thus it is important to stay aware of what those stimuli might be and be ready to recognize the client's reference to them, no matter how coded those references may be.

Perhaps it is not necessary to add that this is one more aspect of therapy that requires a considerable amount of nondefensiveness. If I have made an obvious error, the defensive side of me hopes fervently that it will be overlooked. The client, no more eager to embarrass me than I am to be embarrassed, may try to cooperate. Nonetheless it is likely that sooner or later a reference to my mistake will show up in the client's material. It is equally likely that it will be sufficiently disguised so that it would be easy for me to let it pass and to allow my error to slip into oblivion. But there is therapeutic advantage to my not doing so. Not the least of this advantage comes from providing clients with very likely the first relationship they have ever had in which the other person discusses their own mistakes with the same interest and energy they bring to any other subject.

We have now seen how much emphasis Gill places on helping clients increase both their awareness of the relationship and their willingness to discuss it. But that is not all Gill is concerned with. A major goal of psychodynamic therapy is the recovery of repressed memories. We turn to that now.

The Place of Remembering

If re-experiencing were the only goal, the therapist would only need to encourage an awareness of the relationship. But as we have seen, Gill also believes in (1) the importance of *remembering* and (2) transference as the royal road to that remembering. Just being aware of the feelings toward the therapist, while vitally important, isn't enough. The client must also be helped to see that some part of those feelings is not entirely determined by the realities of the present situation. Certainly in almost all cases they are *partly* determined by the present realities, but seldom entirely. The remaining determinants are the attitudes, the expectations, and the needs that clients bring to the consulting room. The more clients realize how those old forces affect their relationship with the therapist, the more they will come to understand how they shape one's whole life, and, consequently, the less power those ancient forces will have.

Let me illustrate that, and then let's see how Gill talks about this aspect of transference analysis. I gave an illustration earlier:

> **Client:** I was thinking this week that I talk a lot more in here than you do. (*pause*) I really want to know how my boss feels about me. I can't stand this uncertainty.

Gill would now be alerted to the possibility that, in addition to concern about the boss, there is a hidden allusion to the therapist. As we have seen, he would search for this: "That must be difficult." And when the opportunity occurs: "Is it possible that you also have some questions about how I feel about you?" If the client denies this and continues to deny it after some gentle prompting, then either the attempted decoding was incorrect or the resistance was not ready to yield. In that case the therapist would accept the denial and let it pass. But surprisingly often, Gill teaches, the client acknowledges the decode:

> **Client:** Well, I suppose I have been wondering about that. I mean you don't ever say. To tell you the truth I've been thinking lately that you don't seem very interested in me.
>
> **Therapist:** Can you say what gives you that impression?
>
> **Client:** Not really. It's just an idea I had.

At this point Gill's thought-process goes something like this: "I do give him minimal cues, so it's reasonable he would be trying to figure out what I'm up to and how I feel about him. He has to come up with the most plausible hypothesis he can devise. The hypothesis that I don't reveal more because I'm not interested is certainly plausible. However, the exchange between us has been spirited and quite warm for some weeks, so the ambiguities of the situation don't seem sufficient to account for his hypothesis that I'm not interested in him. Thus it's a safe bet that this is a valuable transference issue." If Gill judges this to be a point in the therapy where it is appropriate to help the client look at the transference aspects of the situation, he might do it like this:

Therapist: That's certainly a plausible idea. There are times when I don't talk very much in here, and that could lead you to wonder just how interested I am in you. (*pause*) On the other hand, it seems to me that we have had some warm interchanges recently. That makes me wonder if there aren't other ways you could possibly interpret my manner with you.

Client: I suppose there are.

Therapist: I wonder if there was an earlier time in your life when you feared that somebody important to you wasn't very interested in you.

Now the therapist is in a position to explore some important genetic material and also to help the client see how early experiences influence his contemporary perceptions.

Interpreting Resistance to the Recognition of Transference

In reading this section, it is important to keep in mind that Gill does not follow Freud in thinking of transference as *distortion*.[15] He does indeed agree with Freud's remarkable discovery that we carry with us, as residua of our childhoods, unconscious expectations and unconscious needs, and that these strongly affect the way we see the contemporary world. But whereas Freud went on to argue that sometimes these needs are so strong that we significantly distort our perceptions, Gill thinks of it differently. Gill reasons that we are all continually faced with the necessity of making inferences from inadequate data. We are all continually faced with ambiguous stimuli and ambiguous situations that we must interpret. We deal with these ambiguities by attempting to resolve them in accordance with those unconscious needs and expectations from our childhood. We are not distorting the world; we are trying to arrive at the most plausible construction of it we can, given the ambiguities and given our history.

Gill emphasizes this because he believes that transference interpretations must never carry the implication of put-down. Interpretations experienced as criticism are likely to make even stronger the client's resistance to recognition of transference.

The process illustrated in the last example Gill thinks of as *interpreting resistance to the recognition of transference*. Just as clients are likely to resist awareness of feelings about the therapist, so are they likely to resist seeing that these feelings are transference phenomena.[16] It is unsettling for us to learn that the determinants of our feelings and perceptions are not only what they seem, and so we tend to resist such discoveries. We are likely to resist it even more strongly when the hidden causes come from the most painful and frightening issues of our history. That is why Gill calls this step interpreting resistance.

Gill suggests that there are three ways of interpreting resistance to the recognition of transference: (1) here-and-now interpretation, (2) contemporary life interpretation, and (3) genetic interpretation.

Here-and-now interpretation

The here-and-now interpretation utilizes aspects of the therapy situation to help the client see that a particular response to the therapist is not as inevitable as it seems. These interpretations depend neither on the client's history nor on the client's life outside the therapy situation. The earlier cited illustration of the client who thinks the therapist isn't very interested in him is an example of this. At first it seems to the client that his fears of the therapist's indifference are entirely determined by the realities of the current situation. The therapist reminds him of overlooked events in the therapy to help him see that those realities are subject to other interpretations and thus prepares the way for the client to explore transference determinants.

I once appeared on my analyst's front porch in a snow-storm and found the screen door locked. I had been entering through that door and the wooden one behind it for many months and had never before found either of them locked. I finally got in by ringing the doorbell. Once on the couch I complained bitterly about being locked out. As we will see in a moment, my analyst knew for certain that the door had not been locked at all. Had she been as tactful as Gill, she might have said, "I can certainly understand your feeling terrible about being locked out in the bad weather, and it is plausible that I had locked the door since you had trouble opening it. However, perhaps there are other interpretations. Perhaps the door was just a bit stuck, and instead of forcing it open, you took that opportunity to re-experience some old feelings. You often feel rejected by me." Though less tactful, she did convey that message. I scoffed.

Upon leaving, 50 minutes later, I examined the door carefully. Indeed, the frame had swollen in the wet weather. Further, to my astonishment, there was no lock on the door. In the next session I went seriously to work on my readiness to feel rejected by her.

Contemporary life interpretation

Contemporary life interpretation is one that helps the client see that a particular attitude toward the analyst is similar to attitudes held toward people in the client's present life. In the preceding example my analyst might have said (with complete accuracy), "Shouldn't we perhaps look at how similar these feelings are to those you have about your teachers and classmates? You often feel that they don't 'let you in.'" I would have agreed, and she might then have said, "So perhaps your interpretation of the stuck door, though certainly plausible, was another instance of those feelings of yours."

Similarly, in the case of the client who thought his therapist wasn't very interested in him, the therapist might have said, "Isn't this the way you feel about many people in your life? Perhaps. . . . "

The idea, of course, is that if clients can see that their feelings about the therapist are similar to feelings they often have toward other people, it will help them see that these feelings toward the therapist are in part transference.

Gill doesn't use contemporary life interpretations as much as he does here-and-now ones. He reasons that he can be most effective when the entire situation, including his evidence for transference, is immediately available to both himself and the client.

Genetic Interpretation

The genetic interpretation is one that helps the client see the similarity between feelings toward the therapist and old feelings. The word *genetic* does not refer to how behavior comes from DNA, but rather is used in the sense of "genesis" — that is, how these themes began in the client's life. Let's look at an example:

Therapist: You sound very angry at me. (*The client is silent.*) Are you feeling angry at me today?

Client: Yes, as a matter of fact, I am kind of angry. (*pause*) I just kind of got the idea that you don't approve of me starting this relationship with this new woman I've met. (*pause*) It isn't anything you've said, particularly. I just kind of get that idea. (*pause*)

Therapist: I think we learn a lot from your seeing me that way. You've mentioned to me a couple of times that your mother let you know how much she disapproved of your beginning to go out on dates. (*Client nods.*) I wonder if we're learning here that there was a good deal of buried anger in you back then. Perhaps that's why you're made at me today and why you think I disapprove of your new relationship.

73

The genetic interpretation helps clients learn the extent to which they interpret contemporary reality in the light of their early experiences. To Gill, this discovery is the more powerful for having been made in the transference, where both parties can see it in its entirety.

In classical psychoanalysis *most* transference interpretations were genetic interpretations. These interpretations have great value to Gill as well since, like the classical analysts, he strongly believes in the necessity of clients learning the ancient origins of their contemporary functioning. But Gill cautions against *over*emphasizing genetic interpretations; there is a danger of becoming so occupied with exploring the past that work on the transference is overlooked. Should that happen, we no longer have a re-experiencing therapy.

The Therapist's Contribution to the Client's Experience

There remains one aspect of Gill's notion of transference recognition to be explored. We have seen how Gill views therapy as an interpersonal situation in which the therapist contributes real cues to the client's experience. Inevitably clients perceive these cues and make the most plausible interpretation of them that they can. Equally inevitably this interpretation is significantly shaped by the transference, that is, by the client's long-standing needs and expectations.

Gill reminds us that it does clients a serious disservice to forget that, far from being flawlessly programmed computers, we therapists are imperfect humans giving off a varied assortment of signals of which we can, at best, be only partly aware.[17] Many of these cues stir in clients ideas about how we view them and how we feel about them. As we become increasingly important to them, these ideas attain ever-increasing significance.

When my clients accuse me of inconsistency, it would be tempting to assume that they are merely expressing — at last — pent-up feelings about the inconsistencies of their parents. And, indeed, they often are. But it would be a costly error for me not to look also at the ways in which I have been inconsistent or at least the ways in which I must *appear* inconsistent to my clients.

> **Client:** I think you're very inconsistent sometimes. (*The therapist ponders this a moment and realizes that she greeted the client less warmly today than she sometimes does.*)

> **Therapist:** I wonder if you thought I wasn't as warm to you as I usually am when you arrived today.

> **Client:** That's right. Sometimes you like me, and sometimes you don't. It would be easier for me if you liked me all the time. (*The therapist reflects and realizes that when the client arrived today, she had still been deeply occupied with the preceding client, but that had lasted only a few moments, and at least consciously she had felt perfectly friendly toward the present client when she'd settled down to work with him.*)

> **Therapist:** I think you're quite right that I wasn't as warm as usual when you arrived today. (*pause*) And your interpreting that as indicating I don't like you as much today seems altogether plausible. I can really see

75

how you'd read it that way. (*pause*) I
wonder, however, if you'd considered that
there are other interpretations. Perhaps I
was distracted. So it might be of value to
see why you chose that plausible
interpretation over some other equally
plausible ones.

And the way is opened for exploring transference implications.

Validating the Client's Perception
and Interpretation

The above example illustrates several of Gills' thoughts
about this sort of interaction. First, he thinks it is important
to validate the client's *perception*. This is in clear distinction
to the classical stance, which implies that everything the
client thinks he sees in the therapist is mere transference
and has nothing to do with anything the therapist actually
did. In this case the validated perception is that the therapist
was less warm in her greeting today. Second, the perception
having been validated, it is important for the therapist to
affirm the plausibility of the client's interpretation. In this
case the therapist labels as plausible the interpretation that
she liked the client less today. Third, it is *not* necessary for
the therapist to take a position on the truth of the client's
interpretation. So it was not necessary for the therapist to
confirm or deny that she liked the client less today. Gill
believes that a therapist must *never* deny having such a
feeling. Since the therapist is trying her best to teach the
client the importance of the unconscious, she had better not
put herself in the position of denying that she may be
influenced by something of which she is unaware. In fact,

76

one should probably be cautious about ever adopting a posture of certainty.

Gill is less insistent that confession be avoided, but he is opposed to it. He thinks it seems to ask the client to withhold criticism ("I admit I did it; don't criticize me.") Also, confession deflects attention from the task—that of elucidating the client's feelings and expectations about the therapist. It is enough, Gill thinks, to validate the plausibility of the client's interpretation. We'll look at this issue more closely in Chapter 7.

Sometimes, Gill reminds us, clients have such a strong need to repeat old situations, and their skill at setting up a replay is so great, that they do indeed succeed in getting the therapist to cooperate unwittingly with their transference wishes; that is they successfully induce the therapist to behave in ways that fill their needs or comply with their expectations. In spite of my best intentions, if I am provoked skillfully enough, I may find myself flirtatious or irritable or disinterested. And, however subtly, I may act those feelings out.

Thus, there is another reason for us, as therapists, to pay close attention to what we ourselves do: It enables us to be alert for and aware of our own countertherapeutic attitudes and behaviors, whether they come primarily from our own unconscious needs or primarily from what the client induces us to meet the *client's* unconscious needs. This topic will occupy us at length in Chapter 6.

Summary

We have seen Gill's two kinds of transference interpretation. The first is aimed at helping clients become increasingly aware of their feelings about the therapist, and the second is aimed at helping them see how their old attitudes

77

determine their interpretation of the events of therapy. Gill teaches that the first stages of therapy should be occupied primarily with helping the client increase awareness; only later should the primary emphasis shift to work on transference recognition. Gill offers us a valuable summary of his theory:

> If the therapist operates on the assumption that psychologically determined psychopathology is a matter of interpersonal relations; if he further believes that for purposes of the psychotherapy the most accurately demonstrable pattern of interpersonal interaction is that being enacted between the patient and himself; and if he further believes that the explication of this pattern of interaction will result in the most far-reaching and stable beneficial influence on the patient's patterns of interaction, he will conclude that the elucidation of . . . the patient's experience of the relationship should be his primary goal. In pursuit of this goal he will be alert to disguised references by the patient to his experience of the relationship with the therapist in the here-and-now; he will make such references explicit, ever mindful that he may be mistaken; he will look first for the role which the patient is attributing to him in this experience, and he will attempt to make that explicit in a spirit of seeing the plausibility of the patient's experience even if that experience and the role attributed to him do not agree with what he subjectively considers to be his role.
>
> Only after the patient's experience has been explored from this point of view will he raise questions about possible other interpretations of the ongoing interaction with the goal of elucidating the patient's transference contribution to his experience, . . . [that is, how the patient's experience of the relationship with the therapist] is significantly related to his past. But he will be ever mindful of a temptation on both his part and the patient's to flee to the exploration of the past from the probably more stressful examination of the present, and he will therefore be biased toward attention to the present rather than the past.[18]

Gill's premise is that remembering is not enough. Merely reconstructing the story of the client's life and the reasons for the client's difficulties is not by itself therapeutic. It must be accompanied by an opportunity for the client to re-experience the old impulses in the presence of the new object of those impulses, that is, the therapist. In order for this re-experiencing to be of value, it must be supported and encouraged by the therapist. In the client's past, these impulses were met with a variety of self-serving responses. Being met with nondefensive support and encouragement will be a unique experience for the client, and it is this experience that Gill sees as essential.

The opportunity for re-experiencing is provided for the client by assigning the highest priority to working with the transference. Gill is certainly not opposed to helping clients analyze events in their contemporary life. He would not criticize a therapist, for example, for helping a client deepen her understanding of her relationships at her job or in her family. Nor is he opposed to helping a client understand the effect of his childhood experiences upon his adult functioning, such as seeing how those occupational or familial relationships are affected by his early history. He thinks all of that has a place well-conducted therapy. But he believes that the most effective therapeutic change is brought about by working within the transference, that is, by continually increasing the client's awareness of the relationship.

The reasons for this are clear. First, Gill believes that it is in the clinical relationship that therapeutic re-experiencing is possible; therefore, that is where the greatest therapeutic leverage is to be found. Second, he believes that talking about other relationships and about childhood events, while certainly helpful, puts both therapist and client in danger of being seduced into intellectual formulations that might become more fascinating than useful.

Thus Gill works as much as possible on interpreting resistance to the transference. During the early stages of therapy he is most concerned with helping the client get in touch with the client's feelings and attitudes about the therapist, as well as feelings and attitudes the client thinks the therapist has about him. As therapy progresses, the emphasis gradually shifts to helping the client learn that these feelings and attitudes are not entirely determined by the situation but are in part determined by the client's ancient needs and expectations.

To Gill, there is no possibility of the therapeutic situation being neutral or of the therapist being a blank screen. Attempts to manipulate the situation to make it neutral may only succeed in presenting the client with a cold and unresponsive therapist. Gill encourages therapists to realize that therapy is inevitably an interpersonal situation and thus to permit themselves a good deal of spontaneity. This requires that they remain aware of the cues they give so that they might understand the client's responses.

Therapists are reminded that the client seldom distorts, but is merely trying to explain limited information with the most plausible hypothesis he can devise.

Finally, Gill believes that an effective therapist must demonstrate the utmost respect for the client, a genuine interest in the client's experience of the relationship, and an unflagging nondefensiveness in responding to that experience. To the extent that the therapist manages to demonstrate those attributes, the situation becomes one never before experienced by the client. And to the extent that the clinical relationship becomes unique in those ways, Gill teaches, it becomes a therapeutic relationship.

$$5$$

The Meeting of Psychoanalysis and Humanism

HEINZ KOHUT

H einz Kohut (1913–1981) was an eminent member of
the Freudian establishment; in fact, he had been the
president of the prestigious American Psychoanalytic Association. His training and credentials were impeccable. And
yet for the past ten years his work has been the subject of
one of psychoanalysis' most acrimonious, energetic, and
fruitful controversies. There are those who see him as a
destructive heretic and those who see him as the messiah.
His critics fear that his growing popularity, which is considerable, will undermine the foundations of psychoanalysis. They argue that for decades psychoanalysis has been
fighting a lonely battle against conservative morality, and
here is a renegade from the very heart of their club going
over to the foe and trying to reduce the importance of sex
and aggression in psychoanalytic theory. And equally
costly, they believe, is his softening of the diamond-hard
discipline of psychoanalytic practice by introducing into it

the warm softness of humanism. His most fervent admirers, on the other hand, believe that he led a successful and long-overdue revolt.

This chapter will take the position that he was neither heretic nor messiah, but rather an uncommonly original psychoanalyst who significantly expanded our thinking about human development, psychopathology, and therapy, without taking anything away from the great insights of classical psychoanalytic theory. This is indeed Kohut's position: "It does not indicate any lack of respect for the great explanatory power of the classical formulations, or any lack of appreciation for their beauty and elegance, when I affirm now that it is possible, from the viewpoint of the psychology of the self . . . to enrich the classical theory by adding a self-psychological dimension."[1]

The Beginnings

Kohut traced the beginning of his movement away from standard psychoanalytic technique to an impasse he was at with a female patient. Every session would contain anguished, bitter accusations directed at him. He saw these as resistance, specifically resistance to his interpretations:

> I was inclined to argue with the patient about the correctness of my interpretations and to suspect the presence of stubborn hidden resistances. . . . For a long time I insisted . . . that the patient's reproaches related to specific transference fantasies and wishes on the Oedipal level. . . . She became [even more] violently angry, and furiously accused me of undermining her . . . and . . . wrecking her analysis.[2]

Kohut was convinced that he was dealing with a straightforward Oedipal transference and that his client was experiencing strong alternating feelings of love and hate for him. After getting nowhere with that approach for some time, he stopped arguing with her and started listening. He began to realize that these urgent, persistent demands and accusations were not instances of resistance at all, but rather represented her attempt to show him the reality of her childhood.

The transference had reawakened some of her earliest memories. She had had a depressed and incapacitated mother who had been chronically unavailable to her. She was showing Kohut what that was like by making demands on him that had been unfulfilled in her early childhood. Looked at as the behavior of a grown person, the demands seemed sufficiently excessive and repetitive to justify their being seen as resistance. But looked at as the demands of a young child trying her best to get her needs filled by an unresponsive mother, they could be seen as appropriate and thus extremely valuable for a therapist trying to understand her.

Kohut's Two Questions: Theoretical and Technical

For the next 20 years Kohut pondered two questions: (1) What was it that this woman hadn't gotten from her parents, and (2) what could a therapist do about it? He applied these questions to each client he saw and to his students' and colleagues' clients. His answers to these questions led him to significant divergences from classical psychoanalysis. One of these divergences was theoretical; the other, technical. The theoretical issue need concern us only briefly; the technical issue is crucial to our topic.

The Theoretical Issue

Freud taught that the newborn infant sees the world as undifferentiated from itself. The infant cannot tell that it is separate from the person who holds and feeds it; all of its psychic energy, that is, all desire and frustration, is directed at this undifferentiated self. Freud called this the stage of primary narcissism. Narcissus, as you may recall, was the handsome Greek youth who spent his time gazing lovingly at his own reflection in a pool. Thus the word *narcissistic*, to describe energy directed toward the self.

As the child matures and comes to realize there are other people out there, some portion of the available energy gets directed at those people — first, of course, toward the primary caretaker. Slowly, as the child grows, more and more of the finite amount of available psychic energy is directed at the outside world, and less and less at the self. In Freud's terms, the child grows from a state of narcissism to one of object-relatedness. The more completely this shift is made, the healthier the person. In the fully mature adult there is thus a relatively small amount of energy still concerned with self-issues.

Kohut gradually came to question whether this was the most useful way to view maturation. He proposed instead that there were two parallel lines of development, rather than the single one postulated by Freud. One of these lines was as Freud described: an increasingly differentiated and mature capacity for object relatedness. The other line was the development of the *self*, which, in the healthy individual, goes on throughout a life-time.[3]

The developmental theory of self psychology

In Kohut's view, there are three strong needs that must be fulfilled if the self is to develop fully: the need to be "mirrored," the need to idealize, and the need to be like others.[4]

The need to be mirrored. The first needs to arise are what Kohut called the grandiose-exhibitionistic need. Children need to be shown by one or both parents that they are special, wonderful, and welcome, that it is a great pleasure to have them around. Kohut taught that all this is not learned through anything the parents specifically say or do; rather it is learned through the most subtle of cues: gesture, expression, tone of voice. And presumably this message can be present in varying degrees. To this parental message of delight in the child, Kohut gave the name mirroring. The child looks to the parent for the answer to "Mirror, mirror on the wall, who's the most wonderful of them all?" If, a reasonable percentage of the time, the mirror replies, "You are, my wonderful child," the grandiose-exhibitionistic needs are met.[5]

Now, no parent can possibly be the perfect mirror all the time, and, Kohut says, that's a good thing for the child. Inevitably the parent will sometimes fail to provide adequate mirroring. If that failure doesn't happen too often or too traumatically, it provides the child with an opportunity. Children who have had many, many experiences of being well-mirrored can draw on the memory of those and thus discover an ability to get along without the mirror — at least for a brief time, at least once in a while. And when that happens, they discover that at least for a brief time, at least once in a while, they can be their own mirror. Kohut called this a "transmuting internalization,"[6] by which he meant that children seize the opportunity of the failed mirror to take the mirroring function into themselves and, as a result, change something basic in their *self*. Gradually, over time, as the child grows and develops, these transmuting internalizations add up to one important aspect of a strong and cohesive self. When this happens the grandiose-exhibitionistic needs are no longer primitive. Children who have been well-mirrored no longer ask or care if they are the fairest of them all. They know that they are acceptable, attractive, and likeable people. And they know this reliably, no matter what messages they may get from the outside world. This means that their self-esteem is firmly rooted, presumably forever.

If the parents are too disturbed or too occupied with questions of their own self-esteem, however, the child never gets enough of those early positive messages. The grandiose-exhibitionistic needs are traumatically frustrated and then repressed because it is too painful to be in touch with them when there is no hope of their being gratified.

Psychoanalytic theory teaches that one of the costs of repressing an important need is that the need does not become integrated into the developing personality. The need is walled off from the *ego*, and because the ego is that part of the personality that orchestrates integration and appropriate maturation, the need remains in its primitive form. This is the fate of grandiose-exhibitionistic needs when they are not gratified. The person, then, is likely to suffer from insecurity and feelings of worthlessness, interrupted on occasion by surges of unrealistic grandiosity and, in some cases, maladaptive boasting when these powerful needs for mirroring burst momentarily through the barrier of repression and futilely strive for some crumbs of gratification. Thus a necessary structure of the *self* is stunted.[7]

The need to idealize. A second strong need of the developing self is the need for what Kohut called an *idealized parental imago*. It is important that the child can believe that at least one parent is powerful and knowledgeable. If this need is fulfilled, the child can count on help from that powerful, knowledgeable, and calm person in dealing with an external world too complex for a young person and with internal events too chaotic and frightening for an immature ego.[8]

As in the case of the parental mirror, there must inevitably be parental failures. No parent is omnipotent or omniscient, and from time to time that fact will reveal itself even to a young child. And the child who has had repeated opportunities to identify with power and knowledge, will be able to discover, when the failures come, some power and knowledge of her own. Thus, bit by bit, through the process of transmuting internalization, the child will come to feel confident about being able to cope both with the external world and with inevitable internal conflicts and pressures. This confidence is a key part of the self.

As this part of the self grows and matures through childhood into adolescence and beyond, it develops indispensable capacities. First, it is the repository of the *ideals* by which life is guided. Second, it exercises control over the impulses, enabling one to utilize them rather than being overrun by them. Third, it develops the capacity for self-soothing in times of stress and pain. And finally, Kohut believed, the "higher" aspects of the personality — humor, empathy, creativity, and wisdom — come from a successfully internalized experience of an idealized parental imago.

Here the danger is that the child cannot idealize either parent. It may be that the parents are locked into a pattern of denigrating each other before the child, or it may be that they have such serious behavior problems that it is painfully obvious to the child that they simply are not candidates for idealization. The child will then have no opportunity to develop this part of the self. Kohut taught that when we meet people who seem to have no joy in life, no capacity to be inspired, and not a lot of access to their vitality, we may be seeing evidence that a need for an idealized parental imago wasn't met.

The need to be like others. The third need of the developing self Kohut called the twinship, or alter-ego, need. He thought that children need to know that they share important characteristics with one or both of their parents, that they are not too "different" from the world into which they have been born. If this need is met, the growing person develops a sense of belonging, of communal status. If this need is not adequately met, children are in danger of feeling that in some basic way they are not like other people, that they are somehow strange and don't fit in.[9]

For much of his career, Kohut had thought that the self could most usefully be understood as having only two components — the grandiose-exhibitionistic and the idealized parental imago. He added the twinship need late in his career and consequently wrote less about it. For our purposes, it is enough to note that it's part of the self. It will be helpful to us in understanding certain transferences.

The self

If these three needs are adequately met, the child develops a healthy *self*, which entails high self-esteem, a guidance system of ideals and values, and the self-confidence to develop one's competence. If these needs are not adequately met, the self will have deficits that interfere with healthy development and produce life-problems of greater or lesser severity. He called these problems self-disorders. (It is interesting to note that Kohut believed that if the parents successfully meet the child's needs in just one of the three areas — mirroring, idealizing, or alter-ego — the child will not develop a serious self-disorder, building what Kohut called compensatory structures in the area of the need that was successfully met.[10])

When Kohut began writing about the psychology of the self, he believed that he had found a new way of understanding a single diagnostic group, which had been called the narcissistic disorders: he thought these were the problems arising from an incompletely developed self, and he called only these conditions self-disorders. But by the end of his life he and his co-workers had become convinced that there are few of us who don't have "self" problems of greater or lesser severity, and among people seeking psychological help there are even fewer.[11]

Kohut called his theory of development self psychology, defining the self as the part of the personality that is cohesive in space, enduring in time, the center of initiative, and the recipient of impressions This self is made up of "structures" that result from the transmuting internalizations.[12]

Kohut taught that the development and maturation of the self is a life-long process and that throughout life a person experiences recurring needs for people (Kohut called these people self-objects) who will furnish mirroring experiences, serve as an idealized imago, fill alter-ego needs for belonging. Kohut's theory is a useful balance for those of us who have come to believe (in part from reading too much psychology) that as mature adults we are supposed to do it all on our own, that only the weak *need* people.

The relationship to Freud's theory of development

That, in greatly simplified form, is Kohut's theory of development. Before we move on to consider his clinical theory, we should consider for a moment the relationship of Kohut's self psychology to Freud's theories of psycho-sexual development and psychopathology. It is not within the scope of this book to describe the latter in detail, but since we are working toward an integration of Kohut, Rogers, and Gill, and since Gill's theories of development and psychopathology draw so heavily on Freud, we should ask whether Kohut's conception of the self's development is supplementary to Freud's or opposed to it.

There is currently a popular tradition in American psychology that holds that all the object relations theories, including Kohut's, are irreconcilably opposed to Freud's theories of motivation, development, and psychopathology.[13] Till the last years of his life, Kohut took a different view; he held that he was building on classical psychoanalytic theory, not replacing it. The theory of self-development was not a replacement for the theory of psychosexual development. it was an addition to it.

I think it is helpful to look at Freud's theories as illuminating the effects of one's *intrapsychic* history, and Kohut's theory (as well as those of other object relations theorists) as showing us the effects of one's *interpersonal* history. Each viewpoint makes a unique contribution to our understanding of the client, and each contributes to our understanding of how the client views the therapist. Replaying the Oedipal drama, a client might see the therapist as an object of desire or fear. Or, revealing an unsatisfied wish for an idealized parental imago, the client might see the therapist as the perfect parent. An alert therapist will be prepared to recognize either.

As a matter of fact, the psychoanalysts teach us, any client who gets deeply into therapy is likely to replay some aspect of the Oedipal drama in the transference. According to the psychoanalytic theory of development, the journey through the Oedipus complex is so significant and so fraught with opportunities for serious repressed conflict that it is likely to play a major role in any client's mental life. Similarly, Kohut taught that the needs for mirroring, for twinship, or for finding an idealized person are so ubiquitous that they are likely to appear somewhere in the transference of most clients. It thus seems to me that the theories are compatible, making it possible for us to integrate Gill's and Kohut's views of the clinical relationship. I trust that integration will become clear as we proceed.

We noted earlier that Kohut had been concerned with two questions: What was it that his client hadn't gotten from her parents, and what could a therapist do about it? We have had a glimpse of his answer to the first question. Now let's concern ourselves with the second.

The Technical Issue

If Gill is our spokesperson for a less stoney and formal aura within the psychoanalytic tradition, Kohut, within that same tradition, went a long step further. We will see in a moment that it is seriously inaccurate to accuse him of being nothing but a kindly handholder although kindness is certainly an important part of his therapy. It has been repeatedly observed that Kohut represents a new coming together of the humanistic and the psychoanalytic traditions, and one major reason for this observation is his insistence that therapists be humane.

A corrective emotional experience?

In the mid-1940s a psychoanalyst named Franz Alexander described successful therapy as a *corrective emotional experience*.[14] Alexander believed that the clients had gotten into trouble and sought therapy because the people who raised them had not treated them well. What they needed was someone significant to treat them better, and Alexander proposed to be that someone. For reasons that are not altogether clear, at least not altogether clear to me, the concept of the corrective emotional experience has received a very bad press over the years. Perhaps therapists saw it as implying reassurance at the expense of learning. Perhaps it evoked images of kindly volunteers giving patients milk and cookies. One can understand how therapists might have felt diminished by this image and feared that it didn't give enough weight to the cognitive aspects of their work. After all, they were engaged in deciphering a complex code — that of the unconscious — and helping patients learn through analysis. What's more, many of them, as we have seen, have always prided themselves on being intellectually and emotionally tough. They were certainly not dispensing milk and cookies.

A related objection may have come from the implication that the corrective emotional experience was to be *gratifying*. We have seen that many therapists argue against gratifying a client's needs on the ground that this only prolongs the problem by keeping the client from learning what a hard world this is. Thus they would object to an intentionally warm and supportive experience. The dogged avoidance of providing such an experience presents the client with a frustrating situation. Many schools of therapy acknowledge this cheerfully and say it's all part of the design: No one gives up a familiar old position without being motivated by some frustration. Kohut took another tack and argued that the frustration that comes from a nonempathic therapist is gasoline poured on the fire. The client got into trouble by being raised in this kind of environment, and more of the same isn't going to help much.

However, as we'll see, Kohut acknowledged the need for a certain *kind* of frustration.

With the advantage of hindsight, objections to seeing therapy as a corrective emotional experience seem pretty silly. Ever since Freud discovered that it was not enough merely to tell patients the reason for their trouble, therapists have been providing one or another sort of corrective emotional experience. Nonetheless objections still are raised.

Empathy

And so, wryly accepting that he is courting his colleague's disapproval, Kohut said that it is indeed the task of the therapist to provide a corrective emotional experience, and that the main component of that experience is *empathy*.[15] In Kohut's view, therapeutic empathy is something quite different from milk and cookies: "The best definition of empathy . . . is that it is the capacity to think and feel oneself into the inner life of another person. It is our lifelong ability to experience what another person experiences, though usually . . . to an attenuated degree."[16] To Kohut the first job of all therapists is to open themselves to the empathic experience which permits them to see the world from the client's point of view. The next task is to let the client know that the therapist has indeed succeeded in seeing it from the client's perspective. Probably no therapist would deny the importance of being able to empathize with the client. Kohut's first point of distinction from many other therapists is the amount of emphasis he puts on *letting clients know that you are doing your best to understand the way it looks to them.*

An occupational hazard: being critical

One major implication of this is that being empathic means not telling clients that their point of view is wrong. This idea is crucial to an understanding of Kohut. He observed that many therapists tend to be critical of their clients. One can understand why. In the first place, therapists are only human and are thus given to the whole range of human foibles, including impatience, unconscious aggressiveness, self-protectiveness, sadistic impulses, and power urges. In other words, therapists are subject to all the vagaries of countertransference.

And beside those inevitable dangers, there are theoretical beliefs held by many therapists that can easily slip over into justifications for being critical:

The concepts of resistance and defense. When Freud first described resistance and defense, they were seen as unconscious phenomena protecting the person against what seemed to be real dangers. But years of thinking of clients as people who ask for help and then do everything possible to interfere with the helper's efforts can easily lead a therapist into behaving as though clients are bad children purposefully making life hard for the therapist.

The belief that self-reliance and self-responsibility are necessary for growth. Kohut believed that the culture at large and the psychotherapy community in particular had developed the puritanical view that the only real adults were those who were strong and self-reliant and who, though they enjoyed and appreciated other people, could get along on their own just as well. Therapists can readily slip into a critical stance when confronted with what they perceive to be a client's dependency. This starts with perfectly good will: I really want my clients to achieve independence and self-reliance because I fear that excessive dependency puts them at the mercy of other people's whims. This wish produces subtle exhortations, and before I know it I am being openly critical. I have gotten caught in the value system that says independence statements are good and should be rewarded, while dependency statements are bad and should be "confronted." Now I am just the latest version of the clients' parents and teachers and preachers, telling them they're doing it wrong.

A corollary to this belief in independence is the distaste many therapists feel for statements that portray the client as a victim. Even if we all agree that clients will be better off when they stop seeing themselves this way (and I certainly feel that way about most clients and about myself), Kohut was most emphatic in his position that criticizing such statements only confirms the client's belief about being a victim — now the victim of the therapist's criticisms.

The belief that immature behaviors should not be encouraged. Some of this belief springs from countertransference: Therapists are often offended by a client's primitive expressions of narcissism, such as unmodulated boasting or unmasked fishing for approval. And some of it springs from a theoretical position that holds that the therapist's job is to show the client how immature these behaviors are. According to Kohut, it is not helpful to view these expressions as childish reluctance to give up old gratifications. He asked therapists to see them as welcome indications that the client has not abandoned the hope of having narcissistic needs met. At a deep level, the client understands the necessity for fully expressing these needs in order to complete the healthy development of the self and go on to more mature gratifications. These immature expressions are the signs that the organism has not been killed, that there is still life-energy and the possibility of growth.

The concept of transference as distortion. It is dangerously easy to sound critical when informing clients that they don't see you the way you really are. We are continually reminded by both Gill and Kohut that this is a particularly costly form of criticism, since we are trying our best to help clients feel free to talk about their feelings for the therapist. This is hard enough under the best circumstances; clients needs all the support they can get.

The foregoing is not meant to imply that there is anything wrong with those viewpoints, at least in moderation. Independence certainly has value. Defense and resistance do exist and have to be contended with. There is nothing wrong with our holding these beliefs; the problem is the critical and judgmental mind-set into which these beliefs seduce us. We want clients to reveal themselves to us. If we are empathic, they will gradually come to trust us. If we punish their revelations, we will teach them to suppress any thoughts they have learned will be criticized.

Kohut taught that lack of empathic acceptance from parents drives whole segments of the personality underground. There, they retain their archaic form and are split off from the modulating and maturing influence of the ego. The therapist is not going to help this by repeating the process. Instead, Kohut counseled, it is necessary to create the conditions in which these previously buried aspects of the self can emerge into the light of day and be empathically accepted. As these aspects reach consciousness, the process of integrating them into the adult personality can begin.

Thus Kohut shared Gill's concern that we not tell clients that their experience is wrong. Empathy means letting clients know that they are, perhaps for the first time, truly understood. And it further means letting them know that, also perhaps for the first time, that the way they see the world is not being judged, but accepted as the most likely way for them to see it, given their individual histories.

Does the therapist actually provide the mirror?

Those who accuse Kohut of serving milk and cookies read him as saying that the therapist's job is to correct the deficit in a client who was never adequately mirrored by actually doing the mirroring in therapy, that is, by repeatedly telling clients that they are indeed the fairest of them all — or at least that they're pretty fair. That's a seriously incorrect reading. Kohut thought that such behavior would be countertherapeutic. What he thought *is* therapeutic is to learn carefully how problems stem from the client's childhood, repeatedly communicating that the client's way of being is understood and understandable. (Kohut reminded us never to derogate the client's parents, rather bearing in mind that those parents themselves had parents.) So instead of saying that the client is the fairest, Kohut might say that the client's feelings of worthlessness were altogether understandable given the lack of positive response received as a child. Arnold Goldberg, one of Kohut's closest associates, puts it like this:

> Analysts gratify neither the demands for mirroring archaic grandiosities nor the demands for approval from archaic idealized self-objects. These demands [are] consistently interpreted . . . in a tactful, nonhurtful, nonhumiliating manner. . . . The analyst does not actively mirror; he interprets the need for confirming responses. The analyst does not actively admire or approve grandiose expectations; he explains their role in the psychic economy.[17]

There is something intuitively powerful about this distinction. If my therapist tells me I'm wonderful, I'm glad he thinks so, maybe even very glad, but somewhere I have to wonder if this is nothing but therapeutic technique, if he says this to everyone, and if it really says anything at all about my worth. And even if I were to believe he thinks so, that's not the same thing as *my* thinking so. When I was a child, my parents were essentially the only source of information about the world, and I was a blank slate on which any message might be written. Those conditions no longer exist, and as we all know to our cost from ordinary living, our self-image is likely to be improved only temporarily by having a loved one tell us we're wonderful.

On the other hand, if my therapist really *gets* what it is like inside me and helps me see that I am like this, not because of some inherent badness, but because of the inevitable laws of cause and effect, a different attitude toward myself becomes possible and with it comes the possibility of change.

Kohut put it this way: A crucially important task for an adult is to be able to seek out people (self-objects) who will gratify one's mature narcissistic needs. (You may recall that to Kohut narcissistic is not a derogatory term. Narcissistic energy is a valuable and important part of one's personality.) Once one has found these self-objects, it is important to be able to accept the mature narcissistic gratifications they offer — through mirroring, through being idealized, or through serving as an alter-ego. Those of us with self-disorders, and I think there must be a lot of us, perpetuate our difficulty (1) by not seeking out people who offer these gratifications, (2) by seeking *primitive* forms of these gratifications, or (3) by not being able to accept the mature gratifications when offered. To Kohut, one goal of therapy is to help clients become more and more able to get these needs met.[18] The therapist who, instead, meets those needs, Kohut taught, does not increase the ability of clients to find self-objects on their own.

What sort of frustration is helpful?

We observed that it is generally believed by many schools of therapy that some kind of frustration is necessary to motivate the client to move from the familiar to the new, particularly to the frighteningly new. And we saw that Kohut did not disagree with that, though he was not impressed with the kind of frustration that comes from therapeutic coldness or nonempathic responses. He thought that optimal therapeutic frustration comes from a different source. The most primitive side of clients wants to be gratified *as children*; that is clients want to be hugged, to be told that they're wonderful, to be told that you will protect them, etc. For all the empathy he provided, Kohut did not provide *these* gratifications. In the context of a warm, supportive empathy, this constitutes the optimal frustration, which motivates change and growth.

Let's look at the difference between actually doing the mirroring and empathically communicating to the client that you have grasped the intensity of the need for that mirroring.

Client:　　The people at work don't seem to find me very interesting. I'm beginning to see that no one really wants to spend much time with me or go out to lunch with me or anything like that. The truth of the matter is that I don't think I'm a very interesting person or very attractive, for that matter. (*He stops and looks expectantly at the therapist.*)

It is tempting for some therapists to say at that point, "Well, I find you interesting, and I think you're quite attractive." This is particularly tempting if it's true. So that's one alternative. Another (the classic psychoanalytic) is to remain silent and wait. Kohut advised neither. In order to understand what he recommended, we must keep in mind the extent to which he emphasized that the manner is as important as the words. What follows must be said with warmth and compassion, or else it will be heard as criticism. And Kohut held as his first priority not to be heard as critical.

Therapist:　　(*trying his best to feel inside himself what it would be like to have such experiences*) It must be extremely painful to believe that people don't find you interesting or attractive.

Client:　　(*still expectantly*) It really is.

　　(*It's now inescapably clear that what is wanted is reassurance.*)

Therapist:　　I would think that with that much insecurity about your being attractive and interesting to people, you must have an overwhelming need to know if that's really true and if people do respond to you that way. I think you must often have that need here — to know if I find you interesting and attractive.

Client: It's true. I think about that stuff all the time.

Therapist: That must be very painful.

(Suppose the client isn't willing to let it go at that.)

Client: Well, how about it? Isn't it true that you feel all those things about me, too?

Therapist: I really understand what a major issue this is for you. And I think I can be much more useful to you by helping you learn about this subject than I could by just being one more person with an opinion about you. My opinions are no better than anyone else's. I think my value to you lies somewhere else. This is a hugely important subject for you. We'll do a lot better trying to understand it then we will settling for some momentary reassurance.

Client: It is a big subject. I guess it's the biggest.

Kohut's psychoanalytic critics might cry "foul" here and say that when Kohut's therapist works this way, he has actually answered the question, if not in words, then in manner. By his warmth, his interest, and his concern he has said a good deal about the client's worth. And to this I think Kohut would have replied: "Guilty as charged." The warmth and interest are indeed parts of the corrective emotional experience that Kohut thought therapy must be. And he would have added that this warm and empathic understanding of the hard path the client has walked is utterly different from pronouncing the client the fairest of them all.

Understanding and explanation

Kohut saw therapy as consisting of two components: *understanding* and *explanation*.[19] The first job of therapists is to understand their clients, as deeply and completely as possible. The tool for this understanding is empathy, and the prerequisite is extreme openness. Kohut taught that therapists must be willing to let go of their preconceptions and their theories as they turn their empathic capacity to the client. The task is not to figure out where the client fits into one's theory; the task is to understand the client's experience as fully as possible. Kohut wrote: "If there is one lesson that I have learned during my life as an analyst, it is the lesson that what my patients tell me is likely to be true — that many times when I believed that I was right and my patients were wrong, it turned out, though only after a prolonged search, that my rightness was superficial whereas their rightness was profound."[20] We have seen how Gill's refusal to view transference phenomena as *distortions* leads to considerable respect for the client. Kohut's strong conviction that the client is the expert on himself deepens that respect.

Here, again, Kohut's approach brings humanistic psychology and the psychoanalytic tradition together. Humanistic therapists and group leaders, led by Carl Rogers, have long insisted that the client was the expert on herself.

Traditionally this has been seen as the direct opposite of the psychoanalytic view, with its notions of the unconscious, resistance, and defense, all of which imply that clients know little about themselves. And now here is a psychoanalyst teaching that clients know what they need a good deal better than the therapist, and that the therapist would do well to listen carefully and attempt to empathically grasp the client's experience.

The first task is understanding and conveying one's understanding to the client. Like Rogers before him, Kohut believed that this in itself is therapeutic. If you do nothing but strive for the deepest possible understanding of the client, and if you communicate that understanding, that experience will be life-changing. That seems intuitively correct, doesn't it? Certainly it would be unique in my experience to be with someone whose first priority was to understand the finest details of my experience and to let me know that they had indeed been grasped. Rogers called this feeling prized. It's hard to believe that it wouldn't have a profound effect on my view of myself.

Recently I had to close my office and see clients in a temporary place. One of my clients refused to meet me there because the parking was too difficult. She was angry and contemptuous that I would even ask her to do such a thing. I committed a whole list of Kohut sins. I told her that the parking was no harder there than anywhere else and that I assumed there was something else underlying her anger. She got angrier and angrier and finally I did, too. It escalated into a near-disaster. Kohut would have felt his way into her situation and said with warmth and understanding, "I can really see how upsetting it is for you to have the stability of our seeing each other disturbed. I think that figuring out where you'd park really is difficult, and I think there must be a lot of other upsetting things about our having to see each other somewhere else. And I can imagine some of those other things are even harder to talk about than the parking." Had she then kept the fight going, he might have said, "I think it must be really hard to have this move just laid on you without your having any say in the matter. It must seem like just one more instance where you get pushed around, where decisions get made for you, where you have to take it or leave it. It must be very hard."

Had I done that, I might have made it possible for her to explore other feelings — or I might have failed to do so. But whatever the outcome, she would have felt heard and understood. As it was, I became just one more in a long series of people telling her she was doing it wrong.

Explanation

Understanding in Kohut's view is therapeutic, but only partially so. To Kohut, complete therapy also requires *explanation* — helping clients see that what they do or what they feel or how they are relating to the therapist makes perfect sense, given their life history.

In the previous example, were the therapy far enough along so that I had the information, and if I thought the client was ready for it, Kohut might have wanted me to have gone on to say, "It's very understandable that you have had such a strong response to this change. We know how inconsistent and undependable your father was. You could never count on him for anything. So it makes perfect sense that you would be badly upset by any inconsistency or unreliability in our relationship."

Explanation has three functions:

1. It helps clients see the roots of their behaviors and increase their cognitive understanding of themselves.

104

2. Kohut, like Gill, was a re-experiencing therapist, and we might expect that he saw *relationship* value in the explanation process. Indeed, he did. Explanation deepens the sense of being understood. If my therapist understands how these behaviors came to be, if she understands that I'm not in trouble because of some inherent badness, but because of early experiences, then she understands me, indeed. Understands and accepts me.

3. And to Kohut, who was a relationship therapist, explanation had still another value: Therapist and client are colleagues building an explanatory system; their relationship is at a more complex and mature level than one merely based on empathy. Thus the client learns to relate on a more mature level.

Together, understanding and explanation have many therapeutic values: They create a climate of growth, they increase clients' understanding of their lives, and they put more and more of clients' behaviors under ego control. In addition, they enable the client to build new self-structures.

Transmuting internalizations in therapy

You will recall that in Kohut's theory of development, the structures that make up the self are slowly built through *transmuting internalizations*.[21] When parents are for the most part supportive, as mirrors, idealized imagoes, and alteregos, their inevitable failures give children a chance to provide those functions for themselves. Our clients have gotten into trouble because their parents failed them in some or all of those functions. So the therapeutic task is to give the client a chance to build the structures that weren't built as a child. In Kohut's view, self structures are built in therapy just as they are in childhood. If the therapist is

105

mostly empathic, the conditions are set for structure building. Just as it impossible for a parent to be perfectly understanding, perfectly empathic, all the time, so it is impossible for a therapist to be perfect. Failures are inevitable. The therapist may be in a bad mood or distracted or just miss what the client is saying. And besides, no therapist can be available all the time. Everyone gets sick. Everyone takes vacations. No one is always there to answer the phone. If these failures don't come too often or too traumatically, and if the therapist acknowledges the failure with empathy and without defensiveness, the same opportunity presented by the inevitable failures of a good parent now presents itself. The client discovers an ability to provide some of that nourishing empathy unassisted. Each time that happens, it is a transmuting internalization, and a bit of structure is added to the self. In successful therapy, slowly over time, the structures are built until the original deficits are healed or until adequate compensatory structures have been built. As in Gill's model, nondefensiveness on the part of the therapist is the key to success.

Let's look at how this might work:

Client: I'm really not looking forward to coming here these days.

(Just as in Gill's model, the therapist silently searches recent events to see if this reaction could have been prompted by something the therapist said or did. It's interesting that a classically trained therapist would be more likely to wonder first what material had recently surfaced that was causing the client anxiety. Kohut's first thought would be: "Have I been guilty of an empathic failure?")

Therapist: Can you say more about that?

Client: Not really. I used to look forward to being here, but lately I'm really not looking forward to coming in.

Therapist: It occurs to me that a couple of weeks ago I told you the dates of my summer vacation. I wonder if I wasn't sensitive enough to how that news would affect you.

Client: Well, I think it's true that I have been thinking that there isn't much sense in getting too deeply into anything as long as you're not going to be here.

Therapist: That makes a lot of sense to me. I remember that when you were living with your grandmother, she used to go away without telling you when she'd be back. I remember how distressing that was for you. So it's really understandable that you would be upset about my vacation, particularly since I was somewhat cavalier in the way I told you about it.

It is always tempting to blame the client for one's own failure of empathy. In the incident mentioned a few pages ago, my first response was to feel self-righteous and silently blame the client for insisting on the parking problem, which seemed pretty silly to me. Such defensiveness is always tempting—and it is very costly. In Kohut's model the main advantage of non-defensiveness is that it facilitates clients' capacity to realize that the failure is not theirs, which in turn enables them to provide the missing empathy for themselves and thus begin the process of repairing the self.

As we recall Gill's distinction between the *remembering* and *re-experiencing* schools of therapy, it seems clear that Kohut, like Gill, was strongly on the side of re-experiencing.

Forms of transference

You will recall Freud's observation that the client's view of the therapist is forced into shapes determined by the client's earliest relationships (the client's templates) and is further influenced by the human tendency to repeat certain old patterns (the repetition compulsion). Kohut added another observation: Once clients discover that they have found someone who is willing to listen to them empathically, the old unmet needs awaken. They may see the therapist as someone who can at last meet the old hunger to be mirrored, as someone who can at last be idealized and from whom strength can be drawn, or as someone like the client in some important way, someone whose presence enables the client to feel like a member of the human race. Clients may hold all these views at different times, then settle down to emphasizing one of these.

When Kohut first developed the idea that certain problems arose from an incompletely developed *self*, he saw these problems as distinct diagnostic categories and made the diagnosis by observing the nature of the transference. He said you couldn't really tell if you were dealing with a self-disorder until you had begun the treatment and could see what sort of transference developed. In this early formulation, he thought that the therapy he was recommending was appropriate only for self-disorders and that classical psychoanalysis was still the preferred treatment for the psychoneuroses.

For instance, the angry woman client described at the beginning of this chapter, "self-righteously demanded exclusive attention and reassuring praise — because her phase-appropriate needs for mirroring had not been met by her self-absorbed mother."[22] Kohut considered this a "mirror transference" and, as a consequence, diagnosed her as a "mirror-hungry personality," a form of narcissistic personality disorder.

A client who looked to the therapist to be someone who could be "admired for his prestige, power, beauty, intelligence, or moral stature"[23] he saw as forming an "idealizing transference," which suggested the diagnosis of "ideal-hungry personality," another form of narcissistic personality disorder.

These narcissistic personality disorders are examples of the self-disorders for which he originally thought his therapeutic method was the treatment of choice.

As his work progressed and he began to think that most of us suffer from some degree of self-disorder, he talked less about the need to decide whether a client suffered from a self-disorder or from some other kind of problem; it more and more seemed to him that his therapeutic principles were applicable to a much wider range of human disturbances than he had originally thought.

Few contemporary therapists are likely to use transference content as the sole diagnostic tool. Nonetheless, I think that Kohut's classifications of the transference can be valuable as reminders of some possible things that might have gone wrong in the client's development.[24]

Sometimes a client will begin to tell me what a good therapist I am and how he brags to his friends about me. I used to assume automatically that I was being buttered up to keep me from leading the therapy into dangerous territory, or that the client was expressing a reaction-formation against angry feelings. Kohut taught me to consider the possibility that this is an idealizing transference and that it should be treated with interest and respect. It should also be treated as a strong indication that as a child this client may have had insufficient opportunity to idealize a parent. It is also an indication that he had *some* chance. Had he had none, he would not even have enough hope to try it again in the transference. All of the narcissistic transferences, the mirror transference, the idealizing transference, and the alter-ego transference are extremely positive. They represent clients' hope; they show that they haven't given up trying to get these needs met.

Let's look at some examples. A client spends time expressing in various ways the hope and the belief that he is the therapist's favorite client. The therapist identifies this as a mirror transference and resists all temptation to lead the client to more "mature and realistic" modes of function. The therapist says, in a warm and supportive manner, "It really is important to you that I like working more with you than with anyone else. And it certainly is understandable. We know how many kids there were in your family and how little time your mother had to pay any attention to you, even when you were very young. It's no wonder that you would have a strong need to know you're special."

Male client to male therapist:	Sometimes it's nice just to hang out with you, without saying too much. You're about my age, and sometimes I think we could have been good friends if we'd met some other way. I like it that you smoke a pipe like I do. It's nice just hanging out.

(A classical analyst might see this as a resistance maneuver; i.e., "hanging out" is a good deal safer than talking about possibly dangerous material. The self-psychologist doesn't focus on this perspective. Instead he recognizes it as an alter-ego transference. He lights his pipe and they smoke quietly for a time.)

Therapist: I get it. (*Then after a long pause:*) I remember how you never had much chance to just hang out with your father, how he was always too busy to have time for you. (*Or, if it's earlier in the therapy, and this information hasn't yet appeared:*) Did you have much chance, as a kid, to hang out with your father?

A couple of words are in order about alter-ego transferences. First of all, they are not confined to same-sex therapists. Second, it is characteristic of them, as opposed to the other transference types, that they can be satisfied in silence. Kohut teaches that a child needs to hear from the mirroring parent and the idealized parent. But the alter-ego person, be it parent, grandparent, or someone else, is different. The model for this is a child spending time with the same-sex parent, quietly cooking or doing woodwork or watching television. (It need not be the same-sex parent, but that's the model.)

The importance of revealing one's humanity

We observed in Chapter 1 that the psychoanalytic and humanistic traditions were coming together in ways that presented new opportunities for therapists to combine the power of the psychodynamic theories with the equal power of a truly humane relationship. Kohut's work represents one of the most important forces in that movement. Though a psychoanalyst to the core, as well as a devoted believer in the power of the unconscious and in the importance of analyzing the transference, he was unflagging in his efforts to free therapists from the rigid values of the past — values that have led to countertherapeutic coldness, judgmental behavior, and, perhaps most destructive of all, defensiveness.

He counseled therapists to permit themselves a relaxed and easy-going manner and a good deal of emotional availability. In his final book he says of his liberation: "I have come to feel freer, and, without guilt and misgivings, to show [my clients] my deep involvement and concern via the warmth of my voice, the words that I choose, and other similarly subtle means."[25]

The importance of nondefensiveness

Like Gill, Kohut reminded us that *defensiveness* is one of the therapist's most dangerous enemies. When under attack, he counseled, the first rule is not to fight back. Most of us are too sophisticated to get *caught* doing this. So we fight back with interpretations and subtle accusations of defensiveness and resistance. Kohut thought this is a bad mistake: If we can empathize with clients, we can open ourselves to discovering just how they see us. Of course, it may not coincide with how we see ourselves, but we're not there to empathize with ourselves; we're there to empathize with our clients. And empathizing with clients when they're seeing us in a bad light is very hard — and very therapeutic. Sometimes a client may exaggerate some failure of the therapist's and blow a small error into a major one. It's tempting to criticize the exaggeration, and it's not a good idea. In this situation Kohut would have the therapist say something like this to the client: "I can imagine how upsetting it must be for you to believe that I have made such a serious error." Gill and Kohut are aligned in assigning importance to nondefensiveness. To Gill it is what makes the re-experience different from the original experience. To Kohut it is the necessary precondition for empathy. To both it is indispensable.

Summary

These are the major aspects of the relationship that Kohut thought helpful to the client:

1. The sense of being listened to by someone truly willing to work at understanding them.

2. The sense of having been deeply understood.

3. The sense of having been accepted.

4. Learning the ancient roots of one's difficulties and thus making sense out of them. This is done through the therapist's explanations.

5. Building new self-structures and particularly new structures to compensate for old deficits. These structures are built through transmuting internalizations following empathic failures of the therapist.

I believe that Kohut has done a good deal more than produce a new theory of narcissism and a new technique of therapy, though he certainly gave us both of those. He offered us, I think, a new freedom to relate to our clients with a spirit of friendly and open generosity that many therapists have long felt as their natural way, but a way denied them by the looming conscience of their profession.

6

Countertransference

A client of mine whom I particularly like, and who happens to be a graduate student in psychology, said to me one day, "On Rogers' eight-point empathy scale I'd give you about a *three*." I felt a flush of indignant hurt rush through my body. It lasted only a moment, and then I set to work suppressing it. "This is wonderful," I said to myself. "I've been waiting for the negative transference for months, and here it is."

Deep down, the hurt was still struggling to make itself known.

"I'm the one supposed to be watching the store around here," I said to myself. My defenses won the struggle, the hurt was successfully suppressed, and with relief I re-established my faith in the myth of psychotherapy: *In this room there is one distressed person with problems and one professional who has it all together.*

If you were to ask me if I believe that, that I have it all together, I would honestly assure you that I believe no such thing; I know only too well how untrue that is. Yet, when I'm in the consulting room with the client, I often assume the myth. I do it partly out of the rationalization that this is no time for me to muck around in my own problems; I've got enough to do, trying to understand the client. And I do it partly out of garden-variety defensiveness and narcissism.

115

Now the problem with this, as you have no doubt already seen, is that my indignant hurt is not likely to go away if I just try to ignore it. It's eventually going to cause me trouble, which is to say it's going to cause my client trouble. Perhaps unconsciously I will wait for a chance to hurt my client back, however subtly. Or, more likely, perhaps I will twist myself out of shape trying to show what an empathic therapist I am. Of course, like most of my fellow-therapists, I am too conscientious to do such things knowingly. But I would certainly be likely do them, nonetheless.

Another client, one I saw some years ago, came to see me because of a recurrent need to sabotage himself whenever success seemed imminent. As I listened to his family history, I felt myself particularly moved and saddened by one part of his story. As far back as he could remember, he had been aware that there was something wrong with his younger brother. The latter had a very hard time in school, and it finally became clear to my client that his brother was retarded. It was also clear that his brother was the most loving person he knew and his best friend. My client went on to become a professional with graduate degrees, but in pursuing the advancement of his career, he managed regularly to snatch defeat from the jaws of victory.

As he told me his story, there were many elements that could have been, and later turned out to be, contributions to his rejection of success. But the one that stood out for me was the sad feeling of leaving his beloved brother farther and farther behind. It's not surprising that I focused on this; my younger sister was born severely brain-damaged and has been in an institution most of her life. Among my feelings concerning my sister are a great deal of sadness and also a considerable amount of survivor-guilt.

As I look back on my work with that client, I am grateful that my own conflicts so quickly directed my attention to *his* survivor-guilt, an area that turned out to be very fruitful.

It could have gone another way. I could have easily felt so much unconscious anxiety about having an area of considerable pain stirred up that, in the interests of self-protection, I would have blinded myself to the importance of my client's relationship with his brother.

Two Hidden Dramas

The depth psychologists have taught us that much of what goes on in the minds of our clients — and also of everyone else — is hidden to them. Each person's history, each person's deepest wishes, impulses, and fears, lie out of sight. Nonetheless, they powerfully influence the person's behaviors and conscious attitudes. According to the depth psychologists, this is as true of the therapist as it is of the client. Thus, in addition to the visible, rational relationship transpiring in the consulting room, there are two hidden dramas in complex interaction with each other: that of the client's psyche and that of the therapist's.

We have seen in previous chapters what a leading role the therapist plays in the client's drama. Beginning with the first phone call, the unconscious templates of the client's history shape the events of the relationship and the characteristics of the therapist into a never-ending kaleidoscope of feelings and thoughts about the therapy and the therapist.

A few years after he described the phenomenon of transference, Freud noted that something similar happens in the therapist with regard to the client. To this phenomenon Freud gave the name *countertransference*, and he saw it as an obstacle.[1] His ideal was the absolutely objective observer whose attention hovered evenly over the associations of the client, and whose own concerns and problems were kept far from the consulting room. When this ideal was not achieved, the therapy suffered. Later, some of Freud's followers began to question this view; certainly there were many instances of countertransference that were detrimental to the client and to the therapy, but it also seemed that there were other instances that taught therapists something about the client's problems they could have learned no other way.[2]

That insight led to a new interest in studying countertransference. Gradually it came to be recognized that no matter how much personal therapy therapists had had, no matter how "well analyzed" they might be, it was inevitable that in the consulting room there would be two complex dramas played out, and one of them was going to occur in the unconscious of the therapist. It seemed clear that the more aware the therapist was of this fact, the safer the client would be, and the richer the therapist's sources of information.[3]

Sources of Countertransference

The history of countertransference theory is filled with controversy about how that word should be defined.[4] We will adopt what is now, I believe, the most common usage and consider countertransference to include *all* feelings and attitudes about the client that occur in the therapist. Countertransference responses may be divided into four types:

1. *Realistic responses.* Some countertransference feelings stem from perfectly realistic responses; for example:

The client is a friendly and attractive person, and I feel positive toward her. Any therapist might feel this way, regardless of personal history or conflicts.

The client is belligerent and somewhat threatening. I feel cautious and a bit frightened.

2. *Responses to transference.* Some countertransference feelings are a response to the client's transference; for example:

Acting out a transference, the client is seductive, and I feel excited—or perhaps frightened.

The client is flattering, and I feel inflated.

The client is critical, and I feel threatened.

3. *Responses to material troubling to the therapist.* Some countertransference feelings arise when a client explores an area particularly troubling to the therapist; for example:

The client talks about homosexual anxiety. If I haven't come to terms with my own sex-identity issues, I might well share the client's anxiety.

I am going through a divorce. Hearing of the client's happy marriage, I feel envious.

4. *Characteristic responses of the therapist.* And some countertransference feelings are ones I take everywhere with me; thus, they accompany me into the consulting room, no matter what the client does:

Some male therapists feel more or less competitive with *every* man they meet. Clients are no exception.

119

Some therapists need to be liked or admired by *everyone* they meet. Clients are no exception.

At the beginning of the chapter I described a client criticizing my lack of empathy. My hurt feelings were primarily an instance of the second type: response to transference. They also had some elements of the fourth type: therapist's characteristic response. I don't take well to criticism, wherever it comes from.

My identification with the client with the retarded brother is primarily an instance of the third type: He brought up an area that is conflictual for me. A sensitive therapist without my history could have picked up the brother's importance; then the countertransference would be considered to be of the first type; a realistic response.

My response to being criticized was one that might well have hurt the client. My response to feeling the pain of the damaged sibling was of value to the client. There are, then, two good reasons for paying close attention to these feelings. First, awareness of the countertransference will help us to protect our clients. Second, this awareness will enable us to profit from the insights these feelings can give us about the client.

Useful and Obstructive Countertransference

Heinrich Racker, in his influential book *Transference and Countertransference*,[5] classifies countertransference phenomena as either *useful* or *obstructive*.*

*Actually Racker names useful and obstructive countertransference "concordant" and "complimentary," respectively. These names are confusing if the reader doesn't have a command of object-relations vocabulary, so I'm using "useful" and "obstructive."

Useful countertransference feelings and attitudes are those that an alert therapist succeeds in using to the client's advantage by continuing to observe and ponder them until they become empathic insights. An example is the sadness stirred in me by the story of my client's retarded brother. My hurt feelings about being criticized by the client whom I particularly liked could have been useful countertransference had I accepted them and recognized that they indicated how much he needed to hurt me just then.

An obstructive countertransference phenomenon is any one that is likely to cause trouble. Had I turned the exploration away from the retarded brother out of my own intolerable guilt and anxiety, that would have been an instance of obstructive countertransference.

An important point to note here is that at every moment our deep characterological, habitual responses lie in wait for us, looking for an opportunity to express themselves as countertransference. This is our old friend the repetition compulsion: just like our clients, each of us has a history that is always eager to make itself known. We have seen that the occurrence of this in our clients provides a powerful therapeutic opportunity; in therapists it is a trap to be looked for vigilantly. What kept me from coolly using my hurt feelings as a useful countertransference was the pressure from my life-long fear of criticism. On the other hand, I was able to utilize my feelings about the retarded brother because my sadness and guilt were not strong enough to swamp my empathy and take me off the job.

Obstructive countertransference

Obstructive countertransference phenomena expose us to a number of dangers:

121

1. Countertransference can blind us to an important area of exploration. Or conversely it can cause us to focus on an area that is more *our* issue than the client's.

From time to time the client hints at an emerging sexual fantasy. The therapist has his own anxieties about that aspect of sexuality and successfully keeps himself from seeing its importance to the client.

The therapist has serious unresolved conflicts about her relationship with her mother. She significantly overemphasizes this aspect of the client's dynamics and succeeds in influencing the client to overemphasize it.

2. Countertransference can cause us to use our clients for vicarious gratification.

A therapist with conflicts about his own dependency feelings is in danger of subtly urging the client toward (superficial) independent actions as a vicarious way of trying to overcome his own dependence. This can only result in the client's conflicts becoming more hidden instead of more available. One could imagine this happening in any area that personally troubles the therapist.

Another example is the temptation to urge the client toward more sexual freedom. It is probably true that for many clients increased sexual freedom is a good thing. It is probably also true that many therapists have less sexual freedom than they would wish, and can easily be tempted to deal with that lack vicariously. There are many reasons why a therapist should be *very* cautious about imposing opinions and advice on clients; this is a major one.

3. Countertransference can lead us to emit subtle cues that greatly influence the client. We sometimes forget how important the therapist is to the client. Consciously and unconsciously clients tune their receiver to the therapist. Little is missed, whether it be facial changes, postural shifts, voice tone, or muscle tension. There is no possible way the therapist can (or should!) control all this. The cues will be transmitted, and many of them will be received and interpreted.

If unconsciously I need a certain client (or all my clients!) to like and admire me, however much I may say aloud that I welcome the expression of negative feelings toward me, the client is likely to perceive unconsciously the thousand tiny cues that reveal how I really respond to anger or criticism. Psychologists who study learning phenomena have established that the unconscious reception of such subtle cues can quickly shape a subject's behavior. If I do not find some way to reduce the intensity of that neurotic need, I am in danger of teaching my clients to emphasize their friendly feelings toward me and suppress the not-so-friendly ones.

If I am erotically attracted to a client, I might transmit a host of seductive messages that could, to say the least, leave the client considerably confused about our relationship.

Every client (except one the therapist really doesn't like) probably stirs two competing sets of feelings in the therapist: therapists want to liberate their clients and send them on their way, and they want to keep them dependent. (This ambivalence appears in practically all parents as well.) If they're not vigilant, therapists will find ways to send conflicting cues to their clients.

4. Countertransference can lead us to make interventions that are not in the client's interest.

If I feel wounded by a client, I might, as we have seen, find a way to hurt the client, all the while sincerely believing I am making the best therapeutic move.

If the client's history with his father stirs my own unresolved anger at *my* father, I am in danger of saying critical and angry things about the client's father. Even with the *purest* of intentions, hostile criticism of the client's family is probably not good practice; motivated by countertransference, it can be destructive.

The client speaks mostly trivia. Kohut has taught us how important it is to look past the defensive trivia to the client's fear. The therapist is then in a position to empathize with the client. But if countertransference feelings of irritation and impatience have been stirred in the therapist, it will be tempting to focus on the trivia and miss the underlying fear. Then the therapist's intervention (e.g., "It seems you're avoiding the things that really concern you") will be heard as criticism, and rather than the underlying fear being reduced, it will be strengthened.

5. Countertransference can lead us to adopt the roles into which we are cast by virtue of the client's transference. For historical reasons that need not concern us here, the client's attempt to influence the therapist to accept these roles is called *projective identification*.[6] Projec-

tive identification puts increasing pressure on the therapist to yield to the client's influence and begin acting the part. When the therapist is successfully influenced in this way, it is called *projective counteridentification*, or sometimes *introjective identification*. The pressure can be as intense as hypnotic induction, and after succumbing to the induction and acting out the role, therapists can find themselves as bewildered as if they had just carried out a posthypnotic suggestion.[7]

If a client persistently accuses a therapist of being nonempathic and hostile, pressures will eventually mount in the therapist to treat the client just that way. If he can resist those pressures, the therapist can learn a great deal, from their very intensity, about the client. The danger, of course, is that they will be difficult for any therapist to resist, and if, in addition, there is buried hostility looking for expression, the therapist is likely to give the client a hard time indeed before waking up.

Educated and intelligent and proud of the fact, the client subtly establishes the implication that we are two wise and special people talking it all over. This provides the therapist with a number of unconscious temptations: Playing such a role is easier than doing therapy, and besides the role is flattering. If the therapist accepts the bait, the client has executed an effective defensive maneuver.

The client treats the therapist like a wise elder who understands the world better than the client and whose advice and opinion are very valuable. I hardly need say how tempting this induction can be.

When a client sees the therapist as particularly wonderful, that is, when in the throes of an *idealizing transference*, this puts considerable stress on the therapist's equanimity. Either or both of two temptations are likely to appear: Out of embarrassment the therapist may start making self-deprecating statements, or the therapist, secretly preening, might start acting out the role of super-therapist.

A female client has a strong positive transference, to which her male therapist responds with pleasure and gratification. At a certain point in the therapy, the client's sexual interest in her husband reawakens. The therapist is consciously pleased and sees this as progress. But unconsciously he feels loss, as well as jealousy of the husband. He is likely then to transmit cues of irritation and sulkiness. If she then redirects her energy toward the therapist (perhaps because she has picked up the cues), the latter is likely to feel guilty toward the husband.*

Useful countertransference

Having examined the *dangers* of countertransference, let's now brighten the picture by looking at how countertransference can be beneficial. There is a close relationship between countertransference and empathy. You will recall that we have defined countertransference as *all* of the therapist's responses to the client; thus it follows that all empathy begins with a countertransference response. Let's consider the necessary conditions for the production of

*This example and several others in this chapter have been taken from, or inspired by, Heinrich Racker.[8]

empathy. First, it seems clear that the only countertransference that is a potential generator of empathy is the countertransference stimulated by the client, not one that the therapist takes everywhere. Second, once the countertransference feeling or attitude has arisen, it becomes therapeutic empathy when the therapist can maintain or achieve an *optimal distance* from the feeling. Thus it is crucial that it not be repressed; that will only cause trouble. And it is crucial that it not be permitted to swamp the therapist, either with obstructive impulses (e.g., fighting back) or with burdensome identification (e.g., feeling too sad to be effective). It needs to be held at that distance that permits a *felt* understanding of the client but does not overwhelm the therapist. Let's look at some examples:

A male client says, "I understand that [*the name of another therapist*] left her husband and is with a new man." The (female) therapist feels a surge of excitement. As she examines it, she realizes it comes from the very warm feeling she has for this client. But why would his remark excite her? The thought occurs to her that he might have fantasies about *her* going to a new man. She waits a moment and then asks him if he has any thoughts about the other therapist's new man. Laughing, the client responds, "I wondered if he had been a client of hers." The therapist is now in a position to explore the transference implications of his remark.

A male client speaks of women in ways that the female therapist hears as degrading. After several instances of this, her objectivity erodes, and she finds herself increasingly angry. It occurs to her that the client could not be unaware of the effect such remarks were likely to have on a female therapist or, for that matter, on any woman.

Her anger subsides as she becomes interested in the question of why he would want to offend her and push her away. She now has the information to explore an aspect of the relationship previously hidden to her.

As the client eloquently and dramatically spins out his story, the therapist becomes aware that he is beginning to feel like the audience at a tragic, romantic drama. It isn't just the drama that makes him feel that way. It's also his distinct impression that the client wants nothing from him but his presence as a rapt audience. At first he finds himself enjoying the role. It's easy work, and the client is indeed entertaining. Then slowly he realizes he is feeling lonely and useless. When asked, the client says he is quite satisfied; he really needs to have his story heard, and he greatly appreciates the attentive listening he is receiving. The therapist's feeling of loneliness deepens and becomes somewhat distressing. And then, one day, he is struck with a strong hunch: Is it possible, he wonders, that the client is showing him what it was like for him as a child, that one or both of his parents were so addicted to narcissistic display that the only available role for a child was as a rapt (and terribly lonely) audience? A new way of understanding and exploring the client's pain is opened to him.

For the past few months the therapy has bogged down in the client's resistance. The client reports feelings of anger and mistrust toward the therapist. The impasse seems impenetrable. One day the therapist realizes that her feelings at the very beginning and very end of the hour are different from the discouragement she feels during most of the session. When the client greets her and when he says good-bye, she feels warm and connected to him. This appears to be in marked contrast to his reported anger and mistrust. It begins to seem to her that at the beginning and end of the session she is receiving subtle messages of affection, perhaps of love.

Therapist: I've been feeling a warm connection with you at the beginning and end of our sessions. I wonder if you've noticed anything like that.

Client: Well, sometimes it seems I don't experience being mistrustful till we get settled down.

Therapist: Well, how do you feel toward me when you first come in and we say hello?

Client: (*pondering*) I feel good. I feel like I like you. The mistrust seems to start a bit later.

Therapist: It feels to me at those times that you like me a *lot*.

Client: (*uncomfortably*) That might be right.

Therapist: We've been stuck at a roadblock for some time.

Client: We certainly have.

Therapist: Do you think maybe that's because liking me so much seems dangerous to you?

(*The client is silent, eyes downcast. When he looks up his eyes are filled with tears.*)

129

Therapist: I can certainly understand how scary that is. *(And the impasse is broken.)*

The Therapist's Difficulties

For the therapist, remaining aware of the countertransference is often the most difficult task of all. We want to be objective and neutral. We want our feelings for the client to be our servants, not our masters. We more than *want* that; we demand it of ourselves. We think of ourselves as professionals who keep our desires and anxieties out of our work.

It does not fit my self-image to allow my feelings to be hurt by a client.

It fits it even less to know I want to punish or make love to a client.

I do not like to think of myself as one who finds some clients particularly appealing and some particularly distasteful.

Nor do I like to think of myself as one who can be charmed, repelled, or intimidated out of continuing to steer a steady course.

No matter how much admiration my ego craves in the rest of my life, I expect of myself that where my clients are concerned, I can say with the Buddhists, "Praise and blame are all the same."

But the truth is that I am probably never for a moment free of one or more of those pressures. Much of the time they are mild enough so that even though I am unaware of them, they do no harm. Sometimes I manage to pay attention to them, and then I learn a great deal about my client and our relationship. Sometimes I go to a colleague for help and discover that I am caught by a destructive set of feelings toward the client from which I have to extricate myself, sometimes with great pain and difficulty. And I have to remind myself continually that it simply is not true that there is one person in this room doing transference and one maintaining a firm grip on objectivity and reality.

Concluding Remarks

Of all the reasons for paying attention to the forces of countertransference, probably none is more important than avoiding treating the client in the way that caused the original wounds. We have seen in the preceding chapters the power of the forces that propel the client toward re-creating in the therapy all significant childhood relationships, including those that caused the trouble in the first place. That phenomenon, transference, is one of the most powerful tools the therapist–client team has at its disposal. And we have seen that in order to utilize that tool for the client's growth and liberation, it is essential that the therapist respond to the transference in ways different from the original responses the client received. When my client sees me as a punishing father and resents me accordingly, it is crucial that I don't respond the way the client's father responded long ago. That is a sure way to reopen the wound. And the laws of countertransference dictate that there will sometimes be strong pressures on me to do just that. It will greatly profit my clients if I remind myself at frequent intervals to keep a vigilant countertransference watch posted.

The purpose of increasing one's awareness of counter-transference forces is not to eliminate countertransference. That would be like trying to eliminate the unconscious. It can't be done, nor should it be, since it is the source of empathy. The goal is merely to shorten the time it takes to recognize and resolve a countertransference attitude or impulse. Inevitably, we are going to have a vast array of feelings, wishes, and fears cascade through us in the presence of each client. Inevitably, we will not always be able to identify these at once and use them to increase our understanding of the relationship. And it is probably equally inevitable that from time to time we will get caught in a countertransference that will burden the therapy and set it back. That is all part of the game.

What we *can* work toward is continually shortening the time required to see what we're up to. The more vigilant we become (I would like to say the more *gently* vigilant we become) about our own attitudes, our own feelings and impulses, our own wishes and fears, the more quickly will we be able to turn the countertransference to the therapy's advantage.

7

The Therapist's Dilemmas

There is a question that rises again and again for every therapist: What should I *give* this client at this moment? As we will see, this question leads to some puzzling dilemmas. Nonetheless some answers seem clear. Though we cannot always do all that we expect of ourselves, we have a pretty good idea of some of the things that we *should* give:

We should always give the clients our full attention and energy.

We should make our best effort to *understand* them, which means to understand what they are experiencing at the present moment and to understand the themes of their lives, both apparent and subtle, as they unfold before us.

We should let them *know* that they are indeed with someone who is trying hard to understand them.

We should give them the safety and freedom to reveal anything they wish, without feeling judged.

And we should give them the security of being certain that they are with an ethical professional who knows the boundaries and will not cross them.

Having said that, each of us is left with an extremely difficult question: How much of myself should I reveal to the client?

How much of my personal life do I talk about?

How free am I to tell clients my feelings about them? That is, when I am aware of a countertransference feeling or attitude, do I discuss it?

How am I to communicate warmth and caring?

What do I do when I find myself guilty of a failure of empathy? Do I acknowledge it? Do I say how I feel about it?

These are among the most complex and interesting questions for the next generation of clinicians to explore and expand upon. I daresay no one, including me, really knows the best answers to them. We have seen how puzzled Rogers became trying to figure out just how far genuineness should extend. It seems likely that there will never be firm answers that work for every client and every situation. What seems important is that we think through the implications of each strategy we explore, that we pay attention to the effects on the client, and above all, that we scrupulously consider whether what we do is for the client or for ourselves.

The Conservative-to-Radical Continuum

We can begin to explore these questions by thinking of the possible answers as falling along a continuum from conservative to radical.

At the right end is the classic psychoanalytic position: Therapy is a one-way encounter. The therapist is to lay as low as possible and *give nothing but interpretations*.[1] We have looked at the excesses of this position and found it one that few modern therapists outside the most conservative psychoanalytic institutes would care to adopt. But it has unmistakable advantages. Foremost among these is the protection it affords against the therapist's acting out the countertransference. One of the slogans heard around the Boston Psychoanalytic Institute some years ago was "The analyst's orthodoxy is the patient's protection." There was something to that. Another bit of wisdom passed around that same institute, one I have held dear for years, was "There are only two ways to do real damage to patients: *seducing them* or *punishing them*. If you do neither of those, you can't get into serious trouble." ("Seducing" meant much more than literally seducing them; it meant working to arouse their desire for you, their admiration for you, or their dependence on you. "Punishing" meant anything, however subtle, calculated to hurt them.) We are less likely to let ourselves slip into acting seductively or punitively if we are restrained by stringent guidelines.

This position has the additional advantage of giving the therapist a clear, consistent guideline. You never have to wonder, "Should I answer that question?" "Should I share this feeling?" The answer is comfortably and forever "No!"

At the left, or radical, end of the continuum we'll put the "encounter therapists."[2] Encounter therapy flourished in certain American subcultures during the sixties and seventies. It is much less common now, but it has left its mark. The encounter therapists operate on the principle that the client's problem is inauthenticity and that a completely open relationship will be therapeutic. The encounter is entirely two-way. Encounter therapists reveal every feeling they have about the client and disclose themselves as fully as they expect the client to. The only limits to the depth, breadth, and form of intimacy are those of ethics.

Whatever the excesses of this form of therapy, it too has its advantages. Like classical psychoanalysis, it has the virtue of consistency. The encounter therapist never has to wonder, "Should I"? The answer is always "Yes!" It has another virtue as well: It attempts to be as egalitarian as possible, thus reducing the power imbalance between therapist and client.

Where do the therapists we have considered fall on this self-disclosure continuum? It seems clear that both Rogers and Kohut gradually moved to the left as their careers progressed. Both came to trust their spontaneity and to express their human warmth more and more. But neither was certain about what was the optimal point on the continuum. Gill remains somewhat farther to the right, although his recommendation that therapists permit themselves warmth and spontaneity shows him to be much more liberal than his analytic forebears.

The Dilemmas

Any therapist who does not have the comfort and security of being safely ensconced at either end of the continuum has to face up to the fact that the questions of self-disclosure present real dilemmas. Rogers, Gill, and Kohut are no exceptions. Let's look at the most basic of those dilemmas.

How much should the therapist disclose?

All of our authors are moderately conservative on this point. All take the position that it is most helpful if the therapy is about the client and not the therapist. There is a strong implication in Gill and Kohut that answering personal questions robs the client of an opportunity to explore the feelings and fantasies that gave rise to the question.

A client of mine once became occupied with the question of my sexual orientation, and in session after session asked me to tell him if I was straight or gay. It is a question I sometimes answer, particularly at the beginning of therapy, when the client is trying to decide whether I'm the right therapist. But in this case I decided not to answer the question and told him in as open and friendly a manner as I could muster that I thought it would be better for his therapy if I were not to answer it. He returned to it repeatedly. When the therapy ended he made a special point of telling me that, although it had been frustrating for him, in the final analysis he was glad I had made that choice. It had given him a chance to go progressively deeper into his fantasies about me, into his hopes and fears about me, and into his complex feelings about his own sexual orientation. He thought that, had I answered the question, he would have felt satisfied and dropped the subject with relief, having managed to avoid what turned out to be an important area of exploration.

The opposite point of view, of course, is that an easy, "no big deal" policy of modest amounts of self-revelation tends to demystify the therapist and the therapeutic process and therefore has advantages. It makes the therapist seem more human, and it reduces a bit the painful imbalance of self-disclosure that is entirely one-way. Also, Kohut reminds us that it is always costly to deal the client an unnecessary

137

rejection. In spite of my own preference for the conservative position here, I cannot disagree with that. Each situation is different, and each client probably profits from different approaches to this question.

I have found these guidelines helpful:

1. I try not to make a foolish fetish out of not talking about myself. If a client, on the way out the door, asks in a friendly and casual way, "Where are you going on your vacation?" I tell where I'm going. If the client were then to probe, however ("Who are you going with? Are you married?"), I would be likely to respond, "Ah . . . maybe we'd better talk about that next time."

2. When refusing to answer a question, I try hard not to look like I'm playing "I've got a secret and am therefore one-up on you." I explain as fully as I can why I am taking this stand. If I think the client is frustrated or angered by this, I say I can understand that reaction very well. I am a member of the generation driven wild by the psychoanalyst's silence in the face of any question at all. None of our authors is recommending that we do that to our clients.

Disclosing feelings

As a therapist, I must decide if it's ever helpful to disclose my feelings about the client, and if so, under what conditions.

Positive regard. To Rogers, it was essential that positive regard not only be felt by the therapist, but communicated to the client as well. There is more than one way of doing that.

1. It can be explicitly stated. Therapists do indeed say to clients, "I like you," I love you," "I find you interesting," "I think you're very attractive," "I think you'd be very good at that job," etc.

2. As opposed to what the therapist *says*, positive regard can be implied by the way the therapist *acts* with the client. The way the therapist listens can demonstrate a sincere effort to understand. The quality of the therapist's posture, facial expression, and tone of voice, — all these can communicate that the therapist holds a basic regard for the client that is constant through the vagaries of superficial human changeability.

In trying to decide whether it's best to communicate positive regard by what you say or by what you do, it is worth pondering why it's important to communicate it at all. One reason is that it's probably not possible to form a therapeutic alliance without communicating positive regard. Another reason is that a major therapeutic goal with most clients is the increase of secure self-esteem. Everything the therapist does is ultimately meant to contribute to this, and the communication of positive regard is no exception.

Given that we have at least those two goals, how is positive regard best communicated? Let's look at the problems with saying it explicitly.

There is, first of all, the question of sincerity. A client could be forgiven for wondering if statements of affection and esteem are little more than what therapists say to all their clients. That problem seems lessened when therapists communicate positive regard by what they do and how they do it, rather than by what they say. I confess to a personal prejudice that sometimes words are cheap, and that real regard is communicated by subtle cues and by actual behaviors.

It is a safe bet that when clients ask their therapists, directly or indirectly, if their therapists like them, they are doing a good deal more than asking that question. They are telling their therapists something important about a lack of secure self-esteem. Offering the requested reassurance may provide temporary relief, but it does not address the underlying issue. And the most serious danger of providing that temporary relief is that it momentarily takes the energy out of the client's concern, and a valuable opportunity may be lost: the opportunity for the client to get in touch with the emotions and the memories surrounding this issue.

So if, directly or indirectly, clients raise the question of my feelings about them, I *don't* tell them I like them, love them, or find them interesting. I let them know how strongly I empathize with the importance this topic holds for them. I do my best to give them every chance to explore the hopes, fears, and fantasies that generate such a question, and the feelings evoked by my not answering it. I explain that I believe this exploration can be of great value to them, since it can give them access to the experiences and resulting attitudes that interfere with their self-esteem and that it can ultimately enhance that self-esteem more strongly and more lastingly than could any momentary reassurance from me.

Sometimes, when I have declined, as gently as possible, to answer a question about my feelings toward the client, I feel regretful about having had to decline. At such times I console myself with the knowledge that my clients probably know more about my attitudes toward them than I do, anyway. For months or years they have been watching me, listening to me, gauging my tone of voice, following the changes in my eyes, noticing when I look sad and concerned, and when and how I smile or laugh. I only know my conscious feelings and attitudes; they, I suspect, know much more.

The therapeutic relationship is effective to the extent that clients are relatively free to explore and express their feelings, free of the inevitable concerns that characterize normal social intercourse. When I am trying to tell a friend my feelings, it's hard enough to stay in touch with those feelings and their changes. But that task is made considerably harder by the fact that I have to concern myself with my friend's feelings, too. Everything I say is going to affect my friend, and each of those changes will in turn cause new changes in me. Furthermore, I am likely to censor those feelings that I anticipate will stir something in my friend that I am not willing to deal with. Thus, most non-therapy situations are not calculated to maximize one's abilities to learn about one's feelings and to risk sharing them. The therapeutic situation can be different. Presented not with an array of changeable feelings, but rather with the constancy of the therapist's presence, clients can deal more easily with their own changing feelings.

Further, the therapeutic relationship is unique in that the clients are encouraged to explore the *far reaches* of their wishes, impulses, fears, and fantasies. That implies going beyond what is "realistic" or what is acceptable in a normal relationship. I think that is helped by therapists maintaining a relatively constant posture of accepting, empathic interest and not adding the confusion of their own inevitably fluctuating feelings. Here is an illustration:

Client: I really like you. (*expectant pause*)

Therapist: (*nodding warmly*) I do hear that. (*pause*)
               Can you tell me how you're feeling now?

Client: (*uncomfortably*) It feels bad in a way to say something like that to you and not have you really respond to it.

Therapist: (*nodding*) Can you tell me more about that?

Client: Well, it's not just that I like you. (*pause*) You're very important to me, and I have no idea how you feel about me. It's weird that you're so important to me and for all I know I'm just one more client to you.

Therapist: I can really understand that. It certainly must seem weird, and very frustrating, too. (*pause*) Could you tell me if you have some ideas about how I might feel about you?

Client: You seem very friendly and I guess you like me okay.

Therapist: Sounds like that really isn't enough.

Client: I guess in some ways it really isn't.

Therapist: Could you tell me what *would* be enough?

Client: Oh, I don't know. Maybe nothing would really be enough. I think what I really want is to be the most important person in your whole world. I'd like it if you thought about me when I wasn't here, and if you missed me. I know that's silly, isn't it?

Therapist: It most certainly is not silly. It's very understandable. I can see how important it is to you.

And the way is open for the therapist to empathize and, if it is that stage in the therapy, to help the client see the connection between this need and early deprivations.

Had the therapist responded to the first "I really like you" with "I like you, too," I think it would have been more difficult for this client to become aware of the extremity of his need. It would have seemed to him like a familiar relationship in which two people exchange protestations of affection. And it would have thus seemed inappropriate to explore just how strong the need was.

The existential psychotherapists discuss the pros and cons of explicit statements of positive regard. To them the goal is to enable clients to accept responsibility for their lives, which includes accepting control over their self-image. Therapists don't accomplish this goal by expressing acceptance, love, or admiration for their clients. Indeed, the existential psychotherapists say, such professions could lead to passivity and dependency in clients, reinforcing the belief that self-image is dependent on being admired and accepted by others. Existentialist psychologists do believe however that under certain circumstances a therapist's compassionate acceptance can be the *precondition* for the client's coming to self-acceptance.[3]

This seems to support Kohut's stance of empathizing with the client's need for mirroring, rather than *being* the mirror and saying the client is indeed the fairest of them all. In fact, it may be that Kohut has provided the means whereby the therapist can help the client toward this goal of the existentialists. In order for me courageously to assume responsibility for and control over my self-image (and my destiny as well), perhaps I need to know that someone has really understood the depth of my dependency and has grasped the pain of the early deprivations that generated it.

Let me quickly acknowledge that my position here is controversial. Many wise therapists, certainly including many of Kohut's students, think there are times when it is important to tell clients how much you care for them. These therapists pick such times carefully and speak out only when they think it will evoke a valuable response. Theirs is an entirely defensible position; few rules work every time.

Negative feelings. What do you do about your angry or bored or distant feelings? Do you share those? Rogers and his followers have a clear and convincing position on this question:

1. Do *not* share each passing irritation.

2. Consider sharing a negative feeling only if it is striking or persistent or is interfering with your capacity to be fully present with the client.

3. Before saying it, ask yourself this question: For whom am I doing this? Do I want to say it to unburden myself, to get revenge, to hurt the client? Do I want to say it to show off how authentic I am? If the answer to any of those is yes, keep the feeling to yourself or save it for your supervisor.

4. If it seems to you that your speaking out is indeed meant for the benefit of the client and the movement of the therapy, say it in a manner that shows your basic regard. And say it in a way that minimizes the chance that the client will hear it as criticism. That means taking personal responsibility for what you say. Rogers never says, "I find you boring today." He might say, "I am distressed to find that I am not very interested in our

session today, and it makes me very uncomfortable to tell you this. I think the boredom comes from my not feeling really connected with you. Do you have any idea what's happening between us today that is making me feel this way?"[4]

Empathic failures

What should therapists do when they find themselves guilty of a failure of empathy? Should they acknowledge it? Should they say how they feel about it?

Kohut taught that the therapist's empathic failures are of great value to the client; they are what make transmuting internalization possible. So to begin with, we are certainly to empathize with the client's *experience* of having been mistreated or misunderstood by us, whether or not we think we are guilty. And if relevant, it seems equally non-controversial to follow Gill's advice to validate the perception and affirm the plausibility of the client's interpretation. "I think you're quite right that I wasn't as warm as usual when you arrived today . . . And it seems quite plausible to me that you would interpret that as indicating I don't like you as much today. I can really see how you'd read it that way." Now it becomes controversial: Does one go on to explore whether or not one *is* feeling less friendly toward the client today? Gill's position is clear: the therapist *never* denies a feeling. Knowing that everyone, including every therapist, has an unconscious, the therapist at most admits no *awareness* of such a feeling (if, indeed, the therapist has no awareness of it).

But what if the therapist *is* liking the client less today? Gill's (somewhat tentative) position is that sharing such a feeling is not useful, for reasons examined in Chapter 4. But

145

what is the therapist to do? If, indeed, I am not feeling good about the client, and if I am caught at it long before I have decided it's a feeling worth sharing, is there any honorable, authentic way to avoid dealing with my antipathy? I think not. At this point it must be shared, with all the caution and gentleness that Rogers teaches us.

Now what if I come to think I have made an *error* that has resulted in an empathic failure, such as interrupting or criticizing the client or failing to follow the client's lead? Do I confess the error? Kohut is our most valuable guide here. While he doesn't explicitly deal with this question, his implication is clear: We do whatever maximizes the client's capacity to make use of our failure, whatever will best enable the transmuting internalization to take place. There isn't much doubt that acknowledging the error (without breast-beating) is helpful. Of all the types of self-disclosure we are considering, this seems the one that offers the least costly path to demystifying therapists, thus helping clients develop trust in them. If nondefensiveness is one of the main goals we strive for as therapists, this seems like a good way to practice it.

Stolorow, Brandchaft, and Atwood, innovative students of both Gill and Kohut, introduce a valuable caution into considerations of these questions. They remind us that clients' original wounds came from their caretakers' repeated failures to validate and empathize with their reality. Thus they warn us, whatever choices we make, we must be wary of adopting a stance that seems to bestow on the therapist the prerogative to decide whether the client's psychic reality is indeed *the* reality:

> It is assumed that the patient's experience of the therapeutic relationship is always shaped both by inputs from the analyst and by the structures of meaning into which these are assimilated by the pa-

tient. . . . From this vantage point, the reality of the patient's perception of the analyst is neither debated nor confirmed. Instead, these perceptions serve as points of departure for an exploration of the meanings and organizing principles that structure the patient's psychic reality.[5]

Concluding Remarks

When all is said and done, there may be nothing more important in our work than that we bring as much of ourselves as possible to the therapeutic session. Whether a given feeling or attitude is expressed in words is less important than that we are *present* in the deepest and most complete sense of that word. Understanding this does not resolve the dilemmas of what we should give our clients, but it makes them less intimidating.

I work with students who are having their first experiences as therapists. One of the great satisfactions of this work (both for them and for me) comes at the moment students realize that when they enter the consulting room, they don't need to don a therapist mask, a therapist voice, a therapist posture, and a therapist vocabulary. They don't need to don those accouterments because they have much, much more than that to give their clients.

8

The New Relationship

This book began by noting that for a long time the field of psychotherapy was sharply divided. On the one hand, there were those who received their training from the psychoanalysts and were taught the mysteries of transference along with a somewhat distant attitude toward their clients. On the other hand, there were those trained by the Rogerians and their humanistic descendents, who were encouraged to allow all their natural warmth and compassion into the consulting room but knew little or nothing of the values of working with the transference.

As I suggested in the Introduction, a new harmony, a new consensus, has begun to emerge in the world of the clinical relationship. Some of the old conflicts are beginning to resolve themselves and a cohesive picture is beginning to emerge. Granted, the harmony is not total, and major disagreements will undoubtedly remain. Nonetheless it is an exciting time, one in which ways are being found for integrating the insights of therapists like Rogers and Kohut, whose concerns are for the *human* aspect of the client's experience, with those like Freud and Gill, who maintain a steadfast belief in the power of the unconscious and the therapeutic leverage provided by the transference. In fact, Gill and Kohut themselves have gone a long way toward providing such integration.

The points of view we have studied in the foregoing chapters, when taken together, suggest a way of conducting the clinical relationship. As we have noted, all therapists must develop their own way of working, a way that fits their personality and that honors their accumulating experience. But every therapist needs to start somewhere, and the findings and proposals described in this book provide a good starting place.

An Integration

Let's imagine ourselves therapists who have succeeded in integrating Freud, Rogers, Gill, and Kohut.

We will aspire to *genuineness*. That means we will strive to be transparent, not wearing our therapist mask and not pretending to be who we're not.

And we will remember how important it is to find ways of letting our clients come to know that we consider them worthwhile persons.

We will be nondefensive. Gone forever is the old psychoanalytic fantasy that all the client's responses come *only* from ancient templates. Many of them are perfectly reasonable responses to what the therapist has done or who the therapist is. It is important we are always willing to ask ourselves what we have done to stir up any particular response, and we must always be willing to encourage the client to talk about it.

We will remind ourselves that when clients give us a bad time they may be showing us what kind of bad time someone gave them long ago, and we will do well to stay open to that information.

It is essential that, whatever feelings clients express about us, our response will be interested, encouraging, and without judgment. It is likely that clients have previously gotten very different responses from significant people, and this difference is an important ingredient of the therapy. So whatever the stimulus, we do not preen when praised and do not punish when attacked. And we keep in mind that one of the most costly manifestations of defensiveness is self-justification.

We will allow ourselves a good deal of spontaneity. We will recognize that since we can't possibly be a blank screen, there is no reason to deny our clients our warmth and spontaneity.

We will view our clients with the utmost *respect*. When we think we know better than the clients what they should be doing in therapy, we will seriously consider the possibility that it is they who know better and we will work hard at trying to discover the ways in which they are right. It has been humbling for me to learn from Kohut the extent to which I jump to the conclusion that my client is resisting or defending or acting out. And Kohut also reminded us how important it is to let clients *know* that we see what they're doing in a positive light.

Probably most important of all, is the concept of *empathy*. We get our best information about clients by allowing ourselves to feel what they are feeling, to enter their world as if it were our own. Our empathy is our major therapeutic contribution to our clients.

Thus our job is not to give advice, opinions, or answers, but continually to do our best to *understand* the client. As we saw in the preceding chapter, this means:

151

Understanding what clients are experiencing at this moment, including what they are *feeling* at this moment.

Understanding the gradually unfolding coherence of the themes of their life.

We will let the clients know that we *are* doing our best to understand them. When we don't understand, we'll ask for their help, and when we do think we understand something, we'll tell them that.

It is important to recognize that empathy is not a technique, but an attitude. Beginning therapists are often taught the technique of *reflection*, i.e., saying back to clients what they have just said to you. The hope is, of course, that reflection will convey empathy to the client. ("See, I *am* listening, and I *did* hear what you said.") That's certainly understandable. A therapist needs to say *something*, and reflection is a reasonably safe mode to fall back on when all else fails. There are undoubtedly times when reflection is an excellent way of letting clients know they have been understood and encouraging them to go on. But teaching a technique is probably not the best way to make a therapist empathic.

Therapists needs to learn, not a technique or a group of techniques, but rather ways of opening themselves, first, to their clients' experiences and then to their own spontaneity. That spontaneity will reveal their own special, idiosyncratic way of communicating empathy at that moment.[1]

So we will let our clients know we have *understood*, and then we will find ways to let them know that their feelings are more than just understandable: We will let them know that, given their individual histories, we consider those feelings *inevitable*.

Increasing the Client's Awareness of the Relationship

As therapists integrating the ideas of Freud, Rogers, Gill, and Kohut, we will give our clients a good deal of encouragement to reveal their feelings about us. The transference is where the action is. According to Gill's formula, therapeutic movement results when clients

1. *Re-experience* the ancient thoughts, feelings, and impulses that were originally connected to the genesis of their troubles,

2. Experience those thoughts, feelings, and impulses *in the presence of the person toward whom they are now directed,*

3. *Express* them to that person, and

4. Have that expression met with interest, objectivity, and *acceptance.*

In normal intercourse it is often considered bad form to reveal one's feelings about one's companion. Clients have to learn that it is very good form here. That means encouraging them to talk about their thoughts, feelings, and fantasies about the therapist, as well as their fantasies about the therapist's thoughts, feelings and fantasies. So the therapist will be alert for those opportunities:

If a client says he's afraid that other people will reject him for revealing his true feelings, the therapist will give him plenty of room to explore this fear in his own terms and then wonder (aloud) if he has that fear about her.

If he complains about being surrounded by insensitive people, she will gently wonder if she could be one of those.

If he talks about resenting his boss, after hearing everything he has to say about his boss, she will wonder if this could possibly be a disguised way of talking about her, and, if she sees a way to do it, she will explore that possibility.

And since unremitting respect for the client is one of our guidelines, the therapist will gracefully take "no" for an answer. And when the client does talk about the therapist or acknowledges that the feelings he expresses about the boss may indeed also refer to her, she will accept these statements with empathic interest, and without judgment.

When I first read Gill and set out to encourage my clients to talk more about our relationship, I'm afraid I got carried away. I rather seized them by the lapels at every opportunity and even sometimes when there wasn't an opportunity. If a client spoke of being angry at a lover or afraid of a coworker or dependent on a parent, the words were hardly out of the client's mouth before I was bringing the conversation back to the client and me. It took me a while to discover that this wasn't such a good idea. In the first place, sometimes clients really need time to talk about those outside relationships, and in the second place, my less-than-sensitive precipitousness often failed. After a while I lost some of my new-convert eagerness and settled down to trying to work with a little more restraint and a lot more patience.

I recognized, of course, that clients were concerned with matters other than their relationship with me, and that good therapy would certainly give them an opportunity to work extensively on those other matters. Nonetheless, I continued to believe, and I still believe, that our relationship was the richest therapeutic topic, and that the more time clients spent talking about that relationship, the better off we would be. So I saw myself faced with a new technical problem: How was I to facilitate their talking about their feelings about me? Or how was I to get my client from the lover or boss or parent to me? I began to think of the topic of our relationship as a large, strong fish for which I was angling with a very light line. If I reeled it in too soon or too sharply, I would break the line and lose the fish. If I didn't reel it in at all, I'd never land it. So I learned to give it line and bring it in a little at a time, feeling carefully for what the line would take. I learned to give plenty of attention to *each client's* topic. In the first place, the topic is important to the client. And in the second place, I am fishing with a very light line. Sometimes after I have given a client plenty of line and I feel the line will take it, I reel it in pretty vigorously.

Therapist: (*after a rather full discussion of the client's anxieties about his continuing dependency on his mother*) You know, it occurs to me that it wouldn't be surprising if you had some of those feelings about me.

Client: No, I don't think so. I feel good about our relationship.
(*The therapist's thoughts run something like this: "I do believe in taking 'no' for an answer, and I am reluctant to impose my interpretation on him. Nonetheless some of our recent discussions do make it reasonable to*

155

believe that I might be right about this one. Soon I'll take 'no' for an answer. But not quite yet.")

Therapist: Yes, I hear that. But it would be surprising if other feelings about me and about our relationship didn't crop up from time to time. And I think that it is always helpful if those feelings can be talked about. I'd like to explore this a little further if I might.

Client: Okay.

Therapist: When we started working together, you had some conflict about the very idea of therapy. You thought it was somehow shameful not to take care of your own problems.

Client: I remember that.

Therapist: Lately you've been seeing the value in it and saying that it's become important to you. It would be understandable if those feelings were to stir up some anxiety about getting too dependent on me. Would it be possible for us to explore that?

If that didn't get some kind of affirmative response, I would then let it go and assume that either I was wrong or else that it wasn't yet time for this concern to surface. And, of course, another unsettling possibility is that I just wasn't a good enough fisherman.

Helping the Client Learn About the Power of the Past

Re-experiencing therapists don't believe that, *by itself*, rational understanding will effect much change in the client, and they know better than to get caught in the puzzle-solving game of figuring out and teaching clients how they got that way. Nonetheless they believe it is necessary for clients to understand how their early experiences influence their present lives.

Re-experiencing therapists believe that the transference is the royal road to that understanding. For clients, learning how early experiences affect their relationship with the therapist is a powerful way to grasp just how influential those experiences still are.

Most often, helping the client learn about the power of the past is not the first order of business. With most clients the therapist will spend much of the earlier phases of the therapy just trying to understand their experience and letting them know it has been understood. And the therapist will continually work to increase each client's awareness of the relationship with the therapist. Then, after a time, having begun to gain some understanding of a client and of the themes of that client's life, the therapist will begin helping the client see that reactions to the therapist are inevitably determined *in part* by the attitudes and expectations the client carries everywhere.

The therapist will help clients see that some of their interpretations of events in the relationship, while plausible, are not the only possible ones, and that understanding why they chose those interpretations will teach them a good deal about the influence of the past. The therapist will never imply that the client is *distorting*. Like the rest of us,

157

clients try to make sense out of the available information. So the therapist will validate the client's perception and affirm the plausibility of the client's interpretation.

Becoming increasingly aware of the themes of the client's life, the therapist will be in a better and better position to help the client see that there is nothing "bad" about carrying these attitudes and expectations everywhere. Given the events of the client's life, they are fully understandable, in fact, inevitable.

The Question of Diagnosis

The reader will have noticed that throughout this book the question of diagnosis has not been raised. It seems to me that the question of diagnosis divides therapists into two schools. There are those who, at the beginning of their work with a client, devote a good deal of attention to making a diagnosis. They then set about to shape a style of therapy, including a way of relating, that fits the particular client. The way that these therapists work with a client they have diagnosed as borderline, for instance, is very different from the way they work with a client they consider neurotic.[2] On the other hand, there are therapists who think very little about diagnosis. They do their kind of therapy with whoever comes along. Often these therapists exclude from their practice psychotics, severely retarded clients, and those with serious organic problems. Other than that, they don't concern themselves much with separating clients into categories. However, they make, of course, a continual, moment-to-moment, automatic diagnosis. The way *this* client is at *this* moment determines how such a therapist relates to him or her, and a sensitive therapist relates differently to different clients or to the same client at different times.

The therapists we are considering in this book, Freud, Rogers, Gill, and Kohut, fall into this second school. Rogers, you will recall, is explicit about his view that diagnosis is of no use to a therapist. The psychoanalysts, Freud and Gill, believe that analysis is the treatment of choice of anybody capable of making a genuine relationship with the therapist. Kohut began his study of self psychology with the belief that his therapy depended on an accurate differential diagnosis, but by the end of his life he had changed his mind, believing that all people with emotional problems suffer from deficits of the self and could benefit from his empathic therapy.

Consequently, the approach proposed in this book does not depend on diagnosis (although this style of therapy would be difficult to do with clients in an extreme psychotic condition or with those having serious organic problems). Like all therapy it assumes an attentive sensitivity to each client at each moment and further assumes that therapists' empathy will carefully tune their responses from moment to moment.

Concluding Remarks

All of the therapists whose work we have studied in this book have well-articulated theories of personality, theories of psychopathology, and theories of psychotherapy. Yet as we read them, there emerges the inescapable impression that when they are actually with the client, there is something else as important to them as their theory. That something else is the quality of their presence. When they are at their best, they seem to bring to the client an air of expectant curiosity, a readiness to be surprised, a willingness from moment to moment to have their minds changed. Perhaps empathy, when all is said and done, is putting one's own world aside and fully entering that of the client.

Another characteristic marks our authors: They are remarkably courageous. There are a lot of places to hide in a consulting room; therapists can get through years of work without ever having to learn how a client feels about them or about what they have just said. The therapists we have been studying do their best never to avoid that learning. Indeed, in the case of Gill and Kohut, they court it, believing there is nothing more important that can happen in that room.

At the moment of the existential encounter between therapist and client, the client's whole world is present. All of the clients' significant past relationships, all their most basic hopes and fears, are there and are focused upon the therapist. If we can make it possible for them to become aware of their world coming to rest in us, and if we can be there, fully there, to receive their awareness and respond to it, the relationship cannot help but become therapeutic.

Suggested Readings

On Freud

The best introduction, or reintroduction, to Freud is *Five Lectures on Psychoanalysis*. It can be found in a paperback published by Norton or in *The Standard Edition of the Complete Psychological Works of Sigmund Freud*, published by the Hogarth Press and found in practically every library in the English-speaking world. In the *Standard Edition*, "Five Lectures" will be found in Volume 11, page 3.

Freud's two classic papers on transference are short, and very interesting. They can be found in a paperback collection of Freud's papers called *Therapy and Technique*, edited by Philip Rieff, published by Macmillan's Collier Division. These papers can be found in Volume 12 of the *Standard Edition*, the first, "The Dynamics of Transference," starting on page 99; the second, "Observations on Transference Love," starting on page 149.

On Rogers

Probably the best single introduction to Carl Rogers is his *On Becoming a Person* (Houghton Mifflin, 1961.) I also highly recommend a short paper by Rogers, "The Necessary and Sufficient Conditions of Therapeutic Personality Change," *Journal of Consulting Psychology*. *21* (2) 1957, 95–103. It is said that Rogers considered it his best paper. It certainly is a good one.

An excellent and highly readable text on the Rogerian approach is *Person-Centered Counseling in Action*, by Dave Mearns and Brian Thorne (Sage, 1988). A somewhat less accessible, but very solid and scholarly Rogerian discussion of the clinical relationship is C. H. Patterson's *The Therapeutic Relationship* (Brooks/Cole, 1985).

On Gill

Gill's definitive book on the client–therapist relationship is *The Analysis of Transference*, Volume I (International Universities Press, 1982). Volume 2 of that book, by Gill and Irwin Hoffman, is an extremely valuable series of verbatim transcripts of therapy sessions, annotated to illustrate what the authors consider good and bad instances of the handling of the clinical relationship.

On Kohut

I think the best single book of Kohut's is the posthumously published *How Does Analysis Cure?* (The University of Chicago Press, 1984). It gives a comprehensive picture of his view of therapy and is more easily read than his earlier books. His other two major works, *The Analysis of the Self* (1971) and *The Restoration of the Self* (1977), both published by International Universities Press, are not easy, but they are required reading for anyone wishing to delve deeply into Kohut's thought.

An excellent recent book that gives a clear and complete picture of Kohut's work is *Empathic Attunement: the "Technique" of Psychoanalytic Self-Psychology*, by Crayton Rowe and David MacIsaac (Aronson, 1989).

On Countertransference

Heinrich Racker's *Transference and Countertransference* (International Universities Press, 1968) is still the classic. A very good contemporary book on the topic is *Understanding Countertransference*, by Michael Tansey and Walter Burke (Analytic Press, 1989).

On Existential Psychology

For a rich taste of an existential psychotherapist at work, Irvin Yalom's *Love's Executioner* (Basic Books, 1989) is highly recommended; for a more complete description of existential psychotherapy, you might look at Yalom's *Existential Psychotherapy* (Basic Books, 1980).

All of Rollo May's books are extremely useful for an understanding of the existential perspective. I particularly like *Love and Will* (W. W. Norton, 1969), *Psychology and the Human Dilemma* (D. Van Nostrand, 1967), and *Existential Psychology*, 2nd ed., edited by May (Random House, 1969).

General

Influenced by the work of both Gill and Kohut, in *Psychoanalytic Treatment: an Intersubjective Approach* (Analytic Press, 1987), R. D. Stolorow, B. Brandchaft, and G. E. Atwood add an innovative and extremely useful perspective. An intelligent and searching study of the clinical relationship from a contemporary psychoanalytic point of view is Roy Schafer's *The Analytic Attitude* (Basic Books, 1982), which has become a classic in the field. A fine little book discussing our topic from a Jungian perspective is Mario Jacoby's *The Analytic Encounter* (Inner City Books, 1984).

Notes

Preface

1. Salinger, J. D. (1959). *Raise high the roof beam, carpenters and Seymour, an introduction* (p. 187). Boston: Little Brown.

Chapter 1 Why Study the Relationship?

1. Breuer, J. and Freud, S. (1895). Studies on hysteria. In *The standard edition of the complete psychological works of Sigmund Freud* (Vol. 2, pp. ix–323). London: Hogarth.
2. Freud, S. (1905). Fragment of an analysis of a case of hysteria. In *Standard edition* (Vol. 7, pp. 7–122).
3. Freud, S. (1909). Notes upon a case of obsessional neurosis. In *Standard edition* (Vol. 10, pp. 153–318).
4. Rogers, C. (1942). *Counseling and psychotherapy.* Boston: Houghton Mifflin.
5. Schutz, W. C. (1980). Encounter therapy. In R. J. Corsini (Ed.), *Current psychotherapies.* Itasca, IL.: F. E. Peacock.
6. Gill, M. M. (1982). *Analysis of transference.* New York: International Universities Press.
7. Kohut, H. (1971). *The analysis of the self.* New York: International Universities Press.
8. May, R. (1960). The emergence of existential psychology. In R. May (Ed.), *Existential psychology* (p. 14). New York: Random House.

Chapter 2 The Discovery of Transference: Sigmund Freud

1. Chodorow, N. (1978) *The reproduction of mothering*. Berkeley: University of California Press.
2. Chodorow, N. (1989). *Feminism and psychoanalytic theory*. New Haven, CT: Yale University Press.
3. Freud, S. (1912). The dynamics of transference. In *The standard edition of the complete psychological works of Sigmund Freud* (Vol. 12, pp. 97–108). London: Hogarth.
4. Freud, S. (1920). Beyond the pleasure principle. In *Standard edition* (Vol. 18, pp. v–64).
5. Ibid., p. 22.
6. Freud. The dynamics of transference, pp. 97–108.
7. Freud, S. (1915). Observations on transference love. In *Standard edition* (Vol. 12, pp. 157–171).
8. Freud, S. (1905). Fragment of an analysis of a case of hysteria. In *Standard edition* (Vol. 7, pp. 7–122).
9. Freud, S. (1917). Introductory lectures on psychoanalysis, Lecture XXVII. In *Standard edition* (Vol. 16, p. 436).
10. Freud, S. (1914). Remembering, repeating, and working through. In *Standard edition* (Vol. 12, pp. 145–156).
11. Freud. Introductory lectures, Lecture XXVIII, p. 454.
12. Freud, S. (1940). An outline of psychoanalysis. In *Standard edition* (Vol. 23, p. 177).
13. Freud, S. (1937). Analysis terminable and interminable. In *Standard edition* (Vol. 23, pp. 211–253).

Chapter 3 The Influence of the Humanists: Carl Rogers

1. Rogers, C. (1942). *Counseling and psychotherapy*. Boston: Houghton Mifflin.
2. Rogers, C. R., and R. F. Dymond (Eds.). (1954). *Psychotherapy and personality change*. Chicago: University of Chicago Press.

3. Rogers, C. R. (1957). The necessary and sufficient conditions of therapeutic personality change. *Journal of Consulting Psychology, 21,* 95–103.

4. Rogers, C. R. (1962). The interpersonal relationship: the core of guidance. In C. R. Rogers and B. Stevens (eds.), *Person to person* (pp. 91–92). Lafayette, CA: Real People Press.

5. Ibid., p. 93.

6. Truax, C. B., and Carkhuff, R. R. (1967). *Toward effective counseling and psychotherapy.* New York: Aldine.

7. Rogers. The necessary and sufficient conditions.

8. Rogers, C. R. (1970). *Carl Rogers on encounter groups.* New York: Harper & Row.

9. Rogers. The necessary and sufficient conditions.

10. Rogers, C. R. (1961). *On becoming a person,* pp. 163–182. Boston: Houghton Mifflin.

11. Rogers. The interpersonal relationship, p. 97.

12. Rogers. *On becoming a person,* pp. 184–185.

Chapter 4 A Re-experiencing Therapy:
Merton Gill

1. Gill, M. M. (1982). *Analysis of transference* (Vol. 1). New York: International Universities Press.

2. Gill, M. M. (1982). The point of view of psychoanalysis: energy discharge or person? *Psychoanalysis and Contemporary Thought, 4,* 523–551.

3. Freud, S. (1915). Repression. In *The standard edition of the complete psychological works of Sigmund Freud* (Vol. 14, pp. 143–158).

4. Freud, S. (1926). Inhibitions, symptoms and anxiety. In *Standard edition* (Vol. 20, pp. 77–175).

5. Freud, S. (1940). An outline of psychoanalysis. In *Standard edition* (Vol. 23, pp. 139–207).

6. Freud, S. (1914). Remembering, repeating, and working through. In *Standard edition.* (Vol. 12, pp. 145–156).

7. Freud, S. (1917). Introductory lectures on psychoanalysis, Lecture XXVII. In *Standard edition* (Vol. 16, p. 444).

8. Gill. *Analysis of transference*, p. 44.

9. Ibid., pp. 15–27.

10. Ibid., pp. 64–66.

11. Ibid., pp. 20–21.

12. Ibid., p. 109.

13. Ibid., pp. 86–88.

14. Gill. The point of view of psychoanalysis, p. 543.

15. Ibid., p. 544.

16. Gill. *Analysis of transference*, pp. 107–127.

17. Ibid., pp. 107–114.

18. Gill. The point of view of psychoanalysis, pp. 545–546.

Chapter 5 The Meeting of Psychoanalysis and Humanism:
Heinz Kohut

1. Kohut, H. (1977). *The restoration of the self* (p. 227). New York: International Universities Press.

2. Kohut, H. (1968). The psychoanalytic treatment of narcissistic personality disorders. In P. H. Ornstein (Ed.), *The search for the self* (Vol. 1, pp. 506–507). New York: International Universities Press.

3. Kohut, H. (1971). *The analysis of the self.* New York: International Universities Press.

4. Kohut, H. (1984) *How does analysis cure?* (pp. 192–193). Chicago: University of Chicago Press.

5. Kohut. *The analysis of the self*, pp. 123–124.

6. Ibid., pp. 49–50.

7. Kohut, H., and Wolf, E. S. (1978). The disorders of the self and their treatment: an outline. *International Journal of Psychoanalysis, 59,* 413–425.

8. Kohut. *The analysis of the self*, pp. 7–11.

9. Kohut. *How does analysis cure?*, pp. 198–200.
10. Ibid., p. 99.
11. Ibid., p. 70.
12. Kohut. *The restoration of the self*, pp. 180–184.
13. Greenberg, J. R., and Mitchell, S. A. (1983). *Object relations in psychoanalytic theory*. Cambridge, MA: Harvard University Press.
14. Alexander, F., and French, T. (1946). *Psychoanalytic Psychotherapy*. New York: Ronald Press.
15. Kohut. *How does analysis cure?* p. 78.
16. Ibid., p. 82.
17. Goldberg, A. (Ed.). (1978). *The psychology of the self* (pp. 447–448). New York: International Universities Press.
18. Kohut. *How does analysis cure?*, pp. 76–77.
19. Kohut. *The restoration of the self*, pp. 84–88.
20. Kohut. *How does analysis cure?*, pp. 93–94.
21. Ibid., pp. 70–71.
22. Kohut and Wolf. The disorders of the self, p. 421.
23. Ibid., p. 421.
24. Kohut. *How does analysis cure?*, pp. 193–210.
25. Ibid.

Chapter 6 Countertransference

1. Freud, S. (1910). The future prospects of psychoanalytic therapy. In *The standard edition of the complete psychological works of Sigmund Freud* (Vol. 11, pp. 141–151).
2. Heimann, P. (1950). On countertransference. *International Journal of Psychoanalysis*, *31*, 81–84.
3. Racker, H. (1968). *Transference and countertransference*. New York: International Universities Press.
4. Tansey, M. J., and Burke, W. F. (1989). *Understanding countertransference*. Hillsdale, NJ: Analytic Press.
5. Racker. *Transference and countertransference*.

6. Klein, M. (1946). Notes on some schizoid mechanisms. *International Journal of Psychoanalysis, 33,*433–438.
7. Grinberg, L. (1979). Projective counteridentification and countertransference. In L. Epstein and A. H. Feiner (Eds.), *Countertransference.* New York: Jason Aronson.
8. Racker. *Transference and countertransference.*

Chapter 7 The Therapist's Dilemmas

1. Rangell, L. (1969). The psychoanalytic process. *International Journal of Psychoanalysis, 49,* 19–26.
2. Schutz, W. C. (1980). Encounter therapy. In R. J. Corsini (Ed.), *Current Psychotherapies.* Itasca, IL: F. E. Peacock.
3. May, R. (1958). Contributions of existential psychotherapy. In R. May, E. Angel, and H. F. Ellenberger (Eds.), *Existence.* New York: Basic Books.
4. Rogers, C. R. (1962). The interpersonal relationship: the core of guidance. (C.R. Rogers and B. Stevens (eds.), In *Person to person* (pp. 91–92). Lafayette, CA: Real People Press.
5. Stolorow, R. D., Brandchaft, B., and Atwood, G. E. (1987). *Psychoanalytic treatment: an intersubjective approach.* Hillsdale, NJ: Analytic Press.

Chapter 8 The New Relationship

1. Bozarth, J. (1984). Beyond reflection: emergent modes of empathy. In R. F. Levant and J. M. Shlein (Eds.), *Client-centered therapy and the person-centered approach.* New York: Praeger.
2. Masterson, J. F. (1976) *Psychotherapy of the borderline adult.* New York: Brunner/Mazel.

Index